MICROSCOPY HANDBOOKS 49

Energy-Dispersive X-Ray Analysis in the Electron Microscope

Royal Microscopical Society MICROSCOPY HANDBOOKS

Series Editor

Mark Rainforth (Materials Sciences), *Department of Engineering Materials, University of Sheffield, Sheffield S1 3JD, UK*

Energy-Dispersive X-Ray Analysis in the Electron Microscope

A.J. Garratt-Reed

Center for Materials Science and Engineering, Massachusetts Institute of Technology, Cambridge, Massachusetts, USA

and

D.C. Bell

Center for Imaging and Mesoscale Structures, Harvard University, Cambridge, Massachusetts, USA

© BIOS Scientific Publishers Limited, 2003

First published 2003

Transferred to Digital Printing 2005

A CIP catalogue record for this book is available from the British Library.

ISBN 1 85996 109 6

BIOS Scientific Publishers Ltd
9 Newtec Place, Magdalen Road, Oxford OX4 1RE, UK
Tel. +44 (0)1865 726286. Fax +44 (0)1865 246823
World Wide Web home page: http://www.bios.co.uk/

Distributed exclusively in the United States, its dependent territories, Canada, Mexico, Central and South America, and the Caribbean by Springer-Verlag New York Inc., 175 Fifth Avenue, New York, USA, by arrangement with BIOS Scientific Publishers Ltd., 9 Newtec Place, Magdalen Road, Oxford, OX4 1RE, UK

Production Editor: Eleanor Hooker
Typeset by Saxon Graphics Ltd, Derby

Contents

Abbreviations

AES	Auger electron spectroscopy
CRT	cathode ray tube
EDX	energy-dispersive X-ray
EDXS	energy-dispersive X-ray spectroscopy
EELS	electron energy-loss spectroscopy
EPMA	electron probe microanalysis
ESCA	electron spectroscopy for chemical analysis
ESEM	environmental scanning electron microscope
FET	field-effect transistor
FWHM	full width at half maximum
REELS	reflection electron energy-loss spectroscopy
SDD	silicon drift detector
SEM	scanning electron microscope
STEM	scanning transmission electron microscope
TEM	transmission electron microscope
VP-SEM	variable-pressure scanning electron microscope
WDS	wavelength-dispersive spectroscopy
XPS	X-ray photoelectron spectroscopy
XRF	X-ray fluorescence

Abbreviations

Preface

As we sit at the microscope with users, waiting for data to collect, we frequently find ourselves answering the same questions, time after time. The users need to know what their data tells them about the sample, how it should be interpreted or processed, or a myriad of other details about the experiment. At other times, we find ourselves explaining why a particular experiment cannot be performed, or, at least, why it is more complex than appears at first glance. Sometimes students need help describing these issues to their advisors. Others need the answers to very basic questions like 'My advisor told me to do X-ray analysis in the SEM. What will this tell me about my sample?' And then, again, sometimes we simply discuss the origins of our techniques.

At these times, we have found ourselves wishing for the ideal book to refer them to. We do not need a textbook – good ones have been written, but these users need something simpler and more easily read. Eventually it occurred to each of us, at about the same time, that the way to get exactly the book we had in mind was to write it. We are grateful to our publisher, BIOS, and their reviewers, for agreeing with us, and giving us the opportunity to offer this volume to our colleagues. We hope it is as useful to them as we expect it to be for us!

One does not reach the position of being able to write a book without significant assistance from others. Sometimes it was as simple as a conversation with a colleague in a chance meeting, at other times a result of an organized effort, such as highly productive sabbaticals in Glasgow in 1982 and in Manchester and Liverpool in 1996, and sometimes, again, a result of individual pushing and prodding by collaborators and friends. Although the number of people who contributed in these ways has been huge (some may not even know of their contributions!), AJG-R would like especially to acknowledge Pat Nicholson from Glasgow, Graham Cliff from Manchester and George Smith from Oxford. It was Pat who initially stirred interest in the physics of the generation and detection of the X-ray signals, described in Chapters 2 and 3. Graham's name, of course, has been linked to thin-sample X-ray analysis for nearly three decades, but even in 1996 working with him was a stimulating and exciting experience (unfortunately, ill-health has since forced his retirement). George may be surprised by his inclusion in this list, but without the seemingly endless supply of samples needing analysis that he and others generated, there would have been no point to the rest of the work! George has always known exactly how to challenge us to squeeze that extra bit of information from our micro-analysis, always leading us on to better things. DCB would also like to thank the Characterization Facility at the University of Minnesota, and in particular the director of the lab, Dr Greg Haugstad, and Dr Stuart McKernan for allowing him the time and the encouragement for the pursuit of this endeavour. He must also acknowledge the staff of the electron microscopy lab at MIT who were always encouraging of this goal, Mike Frongillo who always set him straight, Professor Linn Hobbs for providing samples for analysis and critical comments of his research, and of course AJG-R. Our families have also been very patient and supportive with us both. We also must not omit a succession of directors in the Center for Materials Science and Engineering at MIT who have encouraged us and given us the means to pursue this subject. To these, and the many, many other friends and colleagues in the business, we offer our profound thanks.

In thanking Megan Garratt-Reed (AJG-R's daughter) for her help in proofreading the manuscript, we do not in any way abdicate any responsibility for any errors that might persist in the text.

While we hope that our descriptions throughout the book are accurate, they are certainly not rigorous. For readers who are interested in pursuing the subject more deeply, we have provided a bibliography for further reading. Only where we are obviously referring to or quoting from specific pieces of work have we actually provided citations within the text.

Anthony J. Garratt-Reed
David C. Bell
Cambridge, Massachusetts

1 History

Following the discovery of X-rays by Wilhelm Röntgen, at the University of Würtzburg in 1895 (for which in 1901 he was awarded the Nobel Prize), investigations of the properties of this radiation quickly led to new revelations in the physics of matter. Among the better-known scientists, von Laue and then the Braggs (William and Lawrence, father and son, who together won the 1915 Nobel Prize) used X-ray diffraction to investigate the structure of crystalline solids, deriving, amongst other things, a value for inter-atomic distances. Rutherford (winner of the 1908 Nobel prize), who had used various methods to deduce an early version of the nuclear model of the atom, inspired H.G-J. Moseley, working at Manchester University, to use crystal spectrometers to measure the wavelengths of the X-rays emitted by various elemental targets subject to cathode-ray (or, as we would say today, electron) bombardment. This work led to two seminal papers, published in 1913 and 1914, in which he demonstrated what we now know as Moseley's law, which relates the wavelength λ of the principal X-ray line to a new ordinal (which he named the 'atomic number', Z, approximately equal to half the atomic weight) by the relation $\lambda = c/Z^2$, where c is a constant. During his measurements, he had noticed in certain cases when analysing supposedly pure elements that he actually observed X-rays precisely matching those emitted by other elements, and deduced, correctly, that they arose from impurities in his elemental targets. As an afterthought to his work, he added to his first paper the sentence 'The prevalence of lines due to impurities suggests that this may prove a powerful method of chemical analysis'. Surely this was the first reference to the use of electron-induced X-ray emission as an analytical technique. Shortly after writing this, following the patriotic fervour of the time, Moseley enlisted in the British army, and lost his life in action at Gallipoli on 10 August 1915.

As a personal postscript to this short prologue, we will recall that in his later years, when nearing retirement, Sir Lawrence Bragg would travel round Britain to local auditoriums presenting lectures designed to interest school students in physics. Perhaps in at least one of these (in Birmingham, in about 1961) he may have had some success, for among the audience was one of the present authors. Who is to say that this book is not yet another indirect product of the incredibly fertile minds of that group of physicists working nearly a century ago?

It took 35 years for Moseley's suggestion to take a workable form. By 1950, X-ray fluorescence (the excitation of X-rays from the sample by high-energy X-ray bombardment) using crystal spectrometers had become a practical tool, but was limited in its spatial resolution by the impracticability of focusing the incident radiation. In the meantime, transmission electron microscopes (TEMs) had been developed into useful instruments for imaging thin specimens. As a by-product, it became easy to form probes of electrons of the order of micrometers in diameter. It was Raymond Castaing, working in Paris, who put the two together, building his 'Microsonde Electronique' (the first electron microprobe). As part of his work, he formulated the beginnings of what we now know as the *ZAF* correction scheme for quantitative microprobe analysis. Cameca developed his design, and introduced the first commercial electron microprobes.

The limitations on spatial resolution of microanalysis in the microprobe (which we discuss in Chapter 5) were clear at the time. It was Peter Duncumb, working at the Tube Investments Research Laboratory in England who made the first attempt, in his EMMA instrument, to use thin samples. The British firm AEI developed his prototype into a commercial instrument, known as the EMMA-4, introduced in 1969. This achieved its objective of improving the spatial resolution, but at the expense of very limited count rates.

In the meantime, Oatley and his co-workers and students were working on the scanning electron microscope (SEM) in Cambridge. After AEI declined to commercialize the instrument, it fell to Cambridge Instruments to market the first commercial SEM in about 1965. At the time, of course, it was without microanalytical capability.

Energy-dispersive X-ray (EDX) detectors (at least, the lithium-drifted silicon detectors we shall discuss in this volume) were developed during the 1960s, initially for nuclear applications. Application of these detectors to analysis in the SEM in about 1970 was an immediate success, and was quickly followed by their application in EMMA-4 and other TEMs. By 1980, manufacturers had adapted their ranges of SEMs and TEMs to accept EDX detectors and (in the case of TEMs) to form fine probes of electrons and to move towards mitigation of some of the problems, such as contamination and 'hole count' that plagued early TEM microanalysis. During the same period, the use of lanthanum hexaboride (LaB_6) thermionic electron emitters became relatively routine in electron microscopes (previously, the use of thermionic tungsten emitters, of different geometries, had been ubiquitous), and as new instruments were designed, major steps were taken to improve their performance as microanalytical tools. As part of these developments, vacuum improvement became *de rigeur*.

Albert Crewe and his students were working at the University of Chicago, outside the main stream of microscopy development, perfecting the field-emission electron source. It was clear to Crewe that such a source would be of immense value in all areas of application of electron microscopy, and his labours bore fruit in 1970 when his team demonstrated, reliably and reproducibly, the imaging of single thorium atoms attached to strands of DNA. The microscope was a scanning transmission instrument (STEM) seemingly of astonishing simplicity.

Commercialization of the field-emission electron source was not, initially, an unqualified success. Some manufacturers attempted to modify existing columns to take the new gun, and while they did succeed in improving on the performance of the thermionic parent, the overall performance was still compromised. Crewe had approached his work with no preconceptions about microscope design, his background being physics, and it took a new company, VG Microscopes (a subsidiary of Vacuum Generators, in Britain) to follow the same approach to build the first really successful STEM, the HB5, introduced in about 1976. (Some would argue that the instrument was never a commercial success, which may be true, but as a scientific tool, its practical success, with its successors, is undisputed, having set a series of performance benchmarks that other manufacturers are only now drawing close to matching.)

A similar series of missteps bedevilled the initial application of the field-emission gun to the SEM, and it took until about 1990 before researchers began to consider such microscopes to be practical, everyday tools.

In 1980, the use of 30 kV as the acceleration voltage in the SEM would have been considered routine; likewise, use of any voltage above 100 kV in a TEM would have been thought of as a specialized application. Since then, there has been a diverging trend, with the advantages of lower beam energies in the SEM and higher voltages in the TEM becoming apparent. Today, for imaging purposes, the average SEM user will operate at about 5–10 kV, or even lower, while the TEM user will use 200 or 300 kV. As we shall see later in this book, for the microanalyst, the trend in the TEM is an advantage, but in the SEM it poses new challenges.

The X-ray detectors commonly in use today are different only in detail from the detectors used in the early 1970s. It is because of the details, though, including greatly improved resolution, sensitivity to soft X-rays, predictability of characteristics and collection efficiency that EDX analysis in the electron microscope has become an indispensable tool in such a wide range of applications, from production settings to cutting-edge research laboratories.

Before proceeding, it is appropriate to mention acronyms. The title of this book begins 'Energy-Dispersive X-ray Analysis...' – we abbreviate this as 'EDX analysis'. Some other writers use 'EDXS' for 'energy-dispersive X-ray spectroscopy', and others again use 'EDS analysis'. There are references in the literature to 'XEDS' analysis; how the use of this acronym arose we do not know, and we avoid it. It does, though, refer to the same spectroscopy.

2 Principles

2.1 What are X-rays?

X-rays are photons. They have more energy than UV light, and less than gamma rays. Very roughly, the lower energy limit of X-rays is about 10 eV, and the upper limit is 100 keV. X-rays arise in nature as a result of various processes, mainly cosmological. Controlled terrestrial generation of X-rays almost always depends on bombardment of a target (usually metallic) with medium-energy electrons. Two processes are at work. In the first, the atomic electrons are initially excited into higher-energy states by the primary electrons. The excited atoms (strictly, ions) then relax back to their lowest energy state (the 'ground' state), shedding their excess energy in the form of X-rays. Since, as we shall shortly see, the energies of these X-rays are specific to the atom that generated them, they are known as 'characteristic X-rays'. The second process leads to the production of X-rays with a range of energies from zero up to the energy of the primary beam, and for reasons which we shall describe later, they are called 'bremsstrahlung X-rays'.

For X-ray analysis, we depend upon study of the characteristic X-rays; we shall therefore discuss these in some detail next. While the continuum radiation is mainly a nuisance, it must still be understood (and with careful study can indeed provide us clues in interpretation of our spectra); we shall proceed later to discuss its origins.

2.1.1 Characteristic X-rays

Electrons exist in atoms only in specific bound states. The original Bohr model of the atom pictured these as orbits, somewhat like the orbits of the planets bound to the sun by gravity, only the binding force in this case is the electrostatic attraction between the unlike charges of the nucleus and the electrons. Only so many electrons are able to occupy each state for each atom (the specific number depends on the state, but not on the chemical species of atom), and the complement of electrons in a particular state is called a 'shell'. Although we now know the reality to be far more complex, the details are not important for us in this discussion, and the term 'electron shell' is still frequently used to refer to what are more accurately

5

called the 'electron states'. The model provides a remarkably good quantitative fit relating the observed energies of the X-rays (at least of the K-lines) with the atomic number of the element, but again that level of detail will not be needed here.

Since the removal of an electron from the atom requires the expenditure of energy, and since we define the energy of an electron at rest in free space as zero, it follows that the energy of the bound electron is negative; the more tightly bound the electron (that is, the closer the electron is to the nucleus) the more negative – or lower – the energy. The lowest level shell is termed the 'K' shell, the next the 'L' shell, and so on. (This naming convention arose because it was not certain at the time that the K-shell was indeed the lowest – a number of other letters were left in case they were needed.) Because of interactions between the electrons in each shell, they do not all have precisely the same energy – there are actually 'sub-shells' of slightly different energy, except in the K shell. There are three L sub-shells, five M sub-shells, and so on. The energy required to remove the electron from the atom and place it at rest in free space is called the 'binding energy' or the 'ionization energy' (to be really strict, the two terms have different meanings, but for our description we will ignore this).

There are a number of issues that arise because the simple shell model of the atom is modified in solids; although these must be considered when explaining some details of the interaction of electrons with solids, they can, fortunately, be ignored, at least to a first approximation, when discussing electron-induced characteristic X-ray emission (we shall, though, return to this topic in Section 2.5). By way of explanation for any reader who may question this statement, we will mention that almost always in X-ray analysis we are dealing with transitions between relatively tightly bound states, which are the states least affected by chemical bonding or band structure modification effects. We will therefore continue our description as though each atom was in free space.

An incident electron can give enough energy to one of the bound electrons that it is able to leave the atom completely, in a process which is called 'ionization', leaving the now charged atom, or 'ion', in an excited state. For example, if a K-shell electron is removed, the ion has a vacancy now in the K-shell. The ion can go to a lower-energy state if one of the other electrons moves to the K-shell, the excess energy being radiated as the observed X-ray photon. We name the various X-ray transitions by the shell in which the initial vacancy exists; hence an X-ray arising from a K-shell vacancy is called a K X-ray. Clearly, the energy of the X-ray depends not only on the initial vacancy; it also depends on the shell from which the electron originates. The K_α X-ray arises from a transition from the L to the K shell, the K_β X-ray arises from a transition from M to K, the L_α from M to L, and so on. *Figure 2.1* illustrates some of these transitions schematically, using the simple Bohr model. The various sub-shells are accounted for by adding a second numerical suffix, as in $K_{\alpha1}$, $K_{\alpha2}$. This traditional (formally 'Siegbahn') notation for the various transitions is ubiquitously used by analysts, despite the fact that it gets quite complex and confused when dealing with the multiplicity of transitions possible between higher-level shells, and despite the existence of a more descriptive, and simpler notation known as the transition level notation. *Table 2.1* gives the transitions leading to a few of the commonly observed (but not necessarily well-known) X-ray lines.

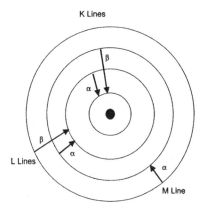

Figure 2.1. Simplified diagram of electron shells, following from the Bohr model of the atom. Some transitions leading to observed X-ray emission are indicated.

Table 2.1. Transitions of a few commonly observed characteristic X-ray lines

Line name	Transition	Line name	Transition
$K_{\alpha 1}$	$L_{III}-K$	$L_{\alpha 1}$	M_V-L_{III}
$K_{\alpha 2}$	$L_{II}-K$	$L_{\alpha 2}$	$M_{IV}-L_{III}$
$K_{\beta 1}$	$M_{III}-K$	L_1	M_I-L_{III}
		$L_{\beta 1}$	$M_{IV}-L_{II}$
		L_η	M_I-L_{II}
		$L_{\beta 4}$	$M_{II}-L_I$
		$L_{\beta 3}$	$M_{III}-L_I$
		$L_{\beta 2}$	N_V-L_{III}
		$L_{\gamma 1}$	$N_{IV}-L_{II}$
		$L_{\gamma 3}$	$N_{III}-L_I$

2.1.2 *Bremsstrahlung*

So far we have discussed only the interaction of the incident electrons with the atomic electrons of the sample. In fact such interactions are relatively improbable. Actually the most probable result of the passage of an incident electron near an individual atom is no interaction at all. Another possibility, also relatively improbable in an individual atom but highly significant when summed over all the atoms of the sample, is the interaction between the incident electron and the atomic nucleus. *Figure 2.2* shows this schematically. Having passed through the screening effect of the bound electrons, the incident electron experiences an electrostatic

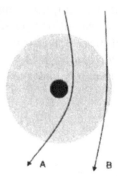

Figure 2.2. Schematic diagram of an electron (A) passing close to the nucleus and suffering significant deflection, and a second electron (B) passing through the outer electron cloud, and being only slightly deflected.

attraction to the positive charge of the nucleus, and is therefore deflected. The closer the electron passes to the nucleus, the greater the deflection. The deflection is (in terms of mechanics) an acceleration of the electron; all charged particles, when accelerated, emit radiation known as 'bremsstrahlung' (a German word meaning 'braking radiation', because the interaction of the electrons and the sample also involves their slowing down), and the photons can have any energy from zero to the energy of the electron beam. These are detected as a continuum in the X-ray spectrum.

The process was examined by Kramers in 1923. He derived an expression relating $B(E)$, the intensity of the radiation as a function of its energy, to Z, the atomic number of the target and E_o, the energy of the incident electron as follows:

$$B(E) = KZ(E_o{-}E)/E \qquad (2.1)$$

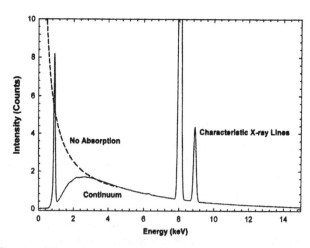

Figure 2.3. Simulated X-ray spectrum as might be observed in a SEM (solid line), with the dashed line indicating bremsstrahlung intensity that would be predicted in the absence of absorption.

where K is the Kramers' constant. While the atomic number Z is seen to be a scaling factor for the intensity, the shape of the function is completely independent of the composition of the target. Since E_0 has to be above the energy of the characteristic X-rays of interest (as we shall see), it is clear that, if the overall X-ray emission is plotted as a function of energy, then the characteristic X-rays are peaks superimposed on slowly varying background of bremsstrahlung, as shown in *Figure 2.3*. For this reason, we often refer to the bremsstrahlung as the 'background', though strictly the background in an observed spectrum also includes components from spurious processes at work in the detector and elsewhere.

Kramers' equation is a good approximation for bremsstrahlung emission in the SEM, but breaks down for higher-voltage (above 100 keV) TEMs. It also ignores more subtle interactions, and better models have been derived, such as the Modified Bethe–Heitler model of Chapman *et al.* (1983), to which we shall refer again in the next section. We may note here that in thin samples, the observed intensity of the bremsstrahlung is a function not only of the atomic number of the sample, but also of the thickness and density.

It would appear from Kramers' equation that the intensity of the bremsstrahlung goes to infinity as the energy approaches zero. Clearly this does not, and cannot, happen. The Kramers equation breaks down at very low energies. Since this part of the energy spectrum is of little value, at least for quantitative analysis (as will be discussed in later chapters), this breakdown is of little consequence.

Unlike the characteristic X-rays, the bremsstrahlung is not emitted isotropically – the intensity is greatest in the 'forward' direction, where we define 'forward' as being in the direction of the incident beam. This is relatively unimportant for SEM work, as the forward direction is into the sample, the electron beam is scattered in all sorts of directions during its propagation through the sample, and the effect is less pronounced in any case for lower-energy electrons. However, in the TEM, there is a significant improvement in the ratio of characteristic to bremsstrahlung intensity as the X-ray take-off angle (defined as the angle between the forward beam direction and the line from the sample to the X-ray detector) is increased. The effect becomes more marked at higher electron beam voltages. Attempts have been made to improve the peak-to-background ratio in the X-ray spectra acquired on TEMs by setting the take-off angle to a large value. However, the compromises that have to be made to fit all the parts in either leads to a very small collection efficiency, or the inability to discriminate between the signal from the sample and spurious events, and so in practice the improvement that was achieved (if any) was more than offset by other problems. Another benefit of higher electron beam voltages, though, is that the overall ratio of characteristic intensity to bremsstrahlung intensity increases; this is realized in practice (although this is only one of several advantages of using relatively high electron voltages in TEMs).

2.2 Ionization cross-section

In Section 2.1 of this chapter, we described how an X-ray is emitted by an atom after an ionization caused by the impact of an incident electron. Since the initial ionization is a prerequisite for the X-ray emission, we will now spend a few paragraphs discussing the process.

The probability of an ionization event occurring is described as a cross-section. The cross-section may be defined as follows.

Imagine an electron beam of unit density – that is, 1 electron per unit area per second – incident on a single atom. If the probability of the atom being ionized in 1 s is expressed as a fraction, then the cross-section is defined as the area represented by that same fraction of the unit area. To use an example: suppose we have an electron probe with a current density of 1 electron per square meter per second (a vanishingly small current – a typical probe can have a density of the order of 10^{25} electrons per square meter per second or more!). It is found that the probability of ionizing the atom is 1 in 10^{28}. The ionization cross-section is therefore 10^{-28} m^2. In atomic physics, cross-sections are more usually measured in units of Barns, where 1 Barn = 10^{-28} m^2. In our imaginary example, therefore, the cross-section is 1 Barn. While the cross-section is expressed in units of area, it is not the same as the 'area' of the atom as 'seen' by the electron beam. It is purely a convenient representation of the ionization probability, which happens to have the dimensions of area.

The ionization cross-section is changed subtly by the chemical bonding states of atoms. Indeed, electron energy-loss spectroscopy is a technique which probes the ionization event in high-resolution detail, and which provides information about the bonding by measuring these subtle changes. However, for X-ray analysis, we are concerned only with the overall probability of generating a vacancy in a particular electron shell. As we have observed before, any chemical effect, if present at all, is so small as to be inconsequential in the vast majority of cases.

An atomic electron cannot be removed from the atom unless it is given at least its ionization energy. Thus, if the energy of the incident electron beam falling on an atom is less than the ionization energy for electrons in a particular shell, the ionization cross-section for that shell will be zero. This, of course, does not imply that less tightly bound shells will not be ionized. For example, while a 5-keV electron beam will not ionize the K-shell electrons in Cu (whose ionization energy is about 8.978 keV), it will most certainly ionize electrons in the L shell, with an ionization energy of 931 eV.

As the energy of the incident electron is increased above the ionization energy, the ionization cross-section increases, quite rapidly at first, until it reaches a maximum at something around three times the ionization energy. After this maximum, the ionization cross-section slowly and monotonically decreases for increasing electron energy. *Figure 2.4* shows a

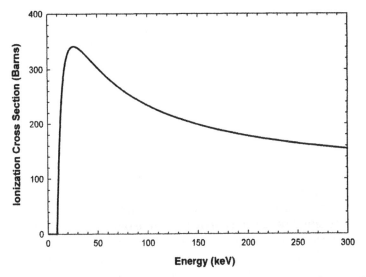

Figure 2.4. Predicted ionization cross-section for K-shell electrons in Cu, as a function of incident electron energy.

plot of a typical ionization cross-section as a function of the incident electron energy.

Ionization cross-sections are extremely difficult to measure. Since knowledge of the cross-section (or at least, how it varies from atom to atom, and with incident electron energy) is an essential requirement for quantitative analysis in the SEM and electron microprobe, a number of authors have proposed parameterized equations, fitted to more or less meagre experimental data, which can then be used to predict the cross-section. While the absolute values of the cross-sections predicted by these different parameterizations can vary, the general dependence of the cross-section on beam energy and target species is reasonably well modelled by most of them. Earlier models ignored any relativistic effects due to the energy of the incident electrons. This was reasonable, as the energies typically employed for SEM and electron probe microanalysis are well below the relativistic range. The same is not true for TEMs working with electron energies above 100 keV, however, and more recent parameterizations include relativistic effects. The data from which *Figure 2.4* was plotted were derived from the relativistically corrected parameterization of Chapman *et al.* (1984), and show the predicted cross-section for the K-shell ionization in Cu. Models for L- and M-shell ionizations are generally considered to be less reliable than models for K-shell ionization, but are still good enough to be useful.

As a very rough generalization, we can say that the most significant determinant of the cross-section, other than the incident beam energy, is the ionization energy of the electron shell. As the ionization energy increases, the cross-section decreases, even if the incident beam energy is increased accordingly. Thus, for example, the ionization cross-section for

Au K-shell electrons at 80.7 keV is 3.15 Barns for 200 keV primary electrons, compared with 327 Barns for ionization of Cu K electrons at 8.98 keV with 20 keV electrons, and 11 208 Barns for Al K electrons at 1.56 keV with 5 keV electrons (all these numbers according to the Chapman *et al.* (1984) parameterization – which we are using here over a wider range than it was originally validated for, but it illustrates the point qualitatively).

When we include the ionization cross-section in equations, it is common to represent it with the symbol 'Q'.

A cross-section for bremsstrahlung generation can be defined in an analogous way. However, since bremsstrahlung can be generated over a range of energies, we can define either a 'total' cross-section – a cross-section for the generation of any bremsstrahlung X-ray – or a 'partial' cross-section – for the generation of a bremsstrahlung X-ray whose energy is within some small range of a particular value (and also, if we wish, travelling at a particular angle to the incident electron direction). Chapman *et al.* (1983) published an equation based upon modified Bethe–Heitler theory (and hence termed the 'MBH' model) which appears to give a good value for the partial cross-section for bremsstrahlung production in most cases of interest to electron microscopists. Since the equation filled more than half a page in their paper, we will not reproduce it here!

2.3 Fluorescence yield

Once an atom is ionized, to be useful to the X-ray spectroscopist, it must decay by the production of an X-ray. Not all excited ions decay in this way. For example, one competing process is the production of an Auger electron, which carries away the excess energy (and which forms the basis of another very useful and widely practised spectroscopy in its own right). Others exist, too. The probability of decay with the production of an X-ray is called the 'fluorescence yield', and varies with the atomic species and shell involved, but not at all with the details of the original ionization event (the energy of the incident electron, or, indeed, whether the event was caused by electron bombardment or some other process), and imperceptibly with the chemical state of the atom.

It might seem to be logical to define a fluorescence yield for each line of a family (for example, the K_α and K_β lines of the K family of X-rays); conventionally, though, this is not done. Instead we define the fluorescence yield for total K-shell (or L-shell, or whichever) X-ray emission, and then take account of the relative probabilities of the different lines within the family with a partition function.

The fluorescence yields for K X-rays are relatively well known; for other shells the knowledge is less complete. In general, it transpires that for low-energy lines, the probability for Auger emission is higher than for X-ray emission, while for high-energy lines, the reverse is the case. Thus, as a general trend, the fluorescence yield increases as the energy of the lines (and, hence, the atomic number of the target atom) increases. Typically the fluorescence yield for K X-rays is in the range of 0.05–0.7, so the probability of an ionized atom emitting an X-ray is reasonably high, although for very light elements the fluorescence yield is far smaller, and for very heavy elements it approaches unity. For C, for example, it is 0.0027, and for Au K X-rays it is 0.9. The fluorescence yield is generally represented by the symbol ω in equations. For the light elements, the product $Q\omega$ is small because ω is small; for the heavier elements, this product is small because Q is small. In the mid-range, covering very roughly the elements Al to Cu, there is a broad maximum, over which the probability of generating K X-rays from atoms of each element does not change by a large amount.

2.4 X-ray absorption

In X-ray analysis we are detecting and measuring X-rays produced within a sample. Before reaching the detector, they must travel through some distance in the sample, and, in most cases, a window in front of the detector. During this passage, they stand some finite chance of being absorbed, with X-rays of different energies having different probabilities of absorption. Thus the measured X-ray intensity is not the same as the generated intensity. In order to derive information about the sample, it is important that the analyst be able to correct for this absorption.

How absorption affects analysis in the SEM and TEM will be discussed in detail in the respective chapters on these techniques. Here we present only a brief description of X-ray absorption.

While X-rays can experience a number of scattering and absorption processes, the only one which causes the X-ray spectroscopist significant concern is photoelectron generation. Photoelectron generation is essentially the same process as ionization of the atom by electron bombardment, only in this case the source of the ionization energy is the incident X-ray, which is completely absorbed, any excess energy being carried away by the ejected electron. (This is the fundamental process employed in yet another important microanalytical technique – X-ray photoelectron spectroscopy, or XPS, also known as electron spectroscopy for chemical analysis, ESCA.) If the X-ray has less energy than the ionization energy of the particular atomic electron, then ionization cannot occur. As the X-ray energy increases, there will be a sudden increase in the ionization probability. In the case of X-ray absorption, unlike with electrons, the probability is maximum if the energy of the incident X-ray is as close as possible to, while remaining above, the ionization energy. For X-rays of still higher energy, the probability falls according to a fairly well defined power law. *Figure 2.5* illustrates a typical relationship.

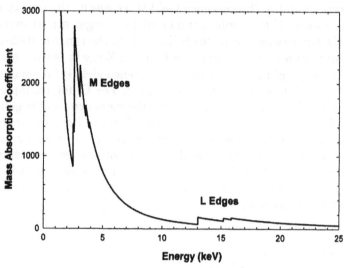

Figure 2.5. Predicted X-ray mass absorption coefficient for Pb, as a function of X-ray energy.

The probability of X-ray absorption is defined in terms of a 'mass absorption coefficient', having dimensions of area/mass (conventionally, cm²/g), and usually represented by the symbol $\frac{\mu}{\rho}$. The X-ray absorption then follows Beers' Law:

$$I = I_0 e^{-\left(\frac{\mu}{\rho}\cdot\rho x\right)} \tag{2.2}$$

where I_0 is the original X-ray intensity, I is the transmitted intensity, ρ is the density of the sample and X is the thickness of material through which the X-rays pass. The mass absorption coefficient is a function of the energy of the incident X-ray and the chemical identity of the absorbing material, but not of the chemical state of the absorber.

As we shall see in a later chapter, knowledge of the mass absorption coefficient is crucial for successful quantitative analysis in the SEM and electron microprobe. Much research has, therefore, been dedicated to its investigation. *Figure 2.5*, which is a plot of the mass absorption coefficient of Pb as a function of energy in the range 100 to 25 keV, is derived from parameterized equations of Heinrich. Such parameterizations are particularly convenient, making it quite easy to compute mass absorption coefficients for absorbers at any desired energy as required, and are discussed further in Chapter 5.

2.5 Insulators, conductors and semiconductors

In order to understand the operation of a solid-state X-ray detector, it is necessary to have at least a basic acquaintance with the band theory of solids. We will now very briefly address this topic.

Electric current is, of course, the movement of electric charge. In a simple monatomic gas, such as helium, the electrons in the He atoms are tightly bound to the nuclei. At room temperature, under the influence of a modest electric field, the He atoms behave as units – the electrons are not separated from the atoms, so, since they remain electrically neutral, they do not respond to the field, and no electric current flows. The gas is an insulator. *Figure 2.6a* is an illustration of the energy levels in such a gas, which is essentially, in modern representation, the old Bohr model.

In a solid, the situation is more complex. The electrons are no longer bound in discrete energy states; rather, the available energies are spread out into ranges, or 'bands' of energy, and particular electrons are not, in general, bound to individual atomic nuclei. However, the laws of physics constrain the total number of electrons that can occupy each band. If a band does not contain all the electrons allowed, then the electrons tend to settle into the lower-energy states. In this case, when an electric field is placed across the solid, the electrons can gain kinetic energy (at the expense of electrostatic potential energy) by moving, in response to the field, towards the positively charged electrode. Likewise, an equal number of electrons will enter from the negative electrode. A current is perceived to flow in the solid. We call it a conductor. This situation is illustrated schematically in *Figure 2.6b*.

If a band contains all the electrons that are allowed, then, when the solid is placed in an electric field, the electrons cannot be accelerated, because doing so would require that they gain energy, but there are no energy states that are allowed in the band for them to occupy. The only way to gain energy is for the electron to occupy a state in a higher energy band – a process analogous to ionization in the gas. In some solids, the lowest allowed energy in the next more energetic band (which is called the 'conduction band') is lower than the highest allowed energy in the fully occupied band (the 'valence band'). In this case, the electric field can accelerate the electrons into the conduction band; the material is a conductor, and is illustrated in *Figure 2.6c*. In most cases, though, the lowest energy in the conduction band is above the highest energy in the valence band. This energy difference is called the 'band gap'. In such solids, if the valence band contains all the allowed electrons (we say that it is 'full'), then it requires that an electron acquire energy at least equal to the band gap before conduction can take place. At low temperatures, the solid does not conduct electricity; it is an insulator. In most insulators, the band gap is many electron volts wide. These materials retain their insulating

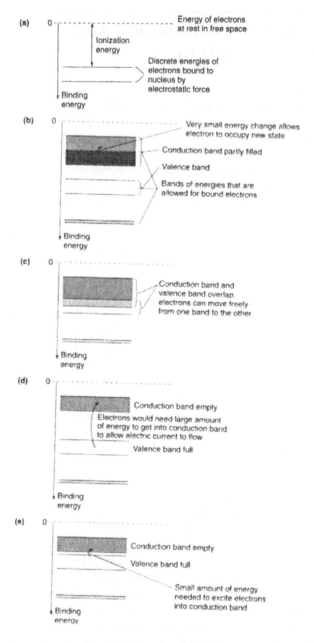

Figure 2.6. (a) Diagram of quantized electron energy levels in a simple gas (such as He). (b) Diagram of energy bands in a typical metal, showing conductivity because of the partly filled band. (c) Diagram of energy levels in some conductors, where the conduction arises because of overlapping bands. (d) Diagram of energy levels in an insulator, in which the valence band is full, the conduction band is empty, and there are, therefore, no available states into which an electron can be excited. (e) Diagram of energy levels in a semiconductor, in which the energy difference (the 'gap') between the valence and conduction bands is sufficiently small that electrons can be excited into conducting states by thermal energy.

properties to very high temperatures. This is the condition illustrated by *Figure 2.6d*.

In a most interesting group of materials, though, the band gap is only a very few electron volts wide, as shown in *Figure 2.6e*. These materials, called 'semiconductors', exhibit many most valuable properties. While, at room temperature, they conduct electricity rather poorly, if a way is found to inject electrons into the structure, these electrons can travel quite freely to the positive electrode, leading to a current flow in the external circuit. (An equivalent process involves removing an electron, creating an electron-vacancy, or 'hole', that behaves in most essential ways like a positively charged electron.) Since the band gap is small, there is a small, but nevertheless significant, chance that electrons may be excited across the band gap by thermal excitation. Hence, depending on the application, it may be necessary to cool the semiconductor to reduce this thermally generated current to an insignificant value. There are a number of materials that display semiconductor properties, of which silicon and germanium are by far the most widely used. Semiconductors must be very pure, as impurity atoms can introduce unwanted electrons or holes, which increase the apparent conductivity of the material. They must also be nearly perfect single crystals, as defects such as dislocations can trap electrons and holes travelling in opposite directions and promote their recombination.

The preceding paragraphs are, of course, a highly simplified summary of the band theory of solids; they do, however, give us the insight we will need to understand the operation of an X-ray detector. We will undertake that discussion in the next chapter.

3 The energy-dispersive X-ray detector

3.1 Introduction

There are several different types of EDX detectors. In this chapter we shall discuss at length only those types that are commonly used on electron microscopes, namely the lithium-drifted silicon (or Si(Li)) detector, and its close cousin, the high-purity germanium (HPGe) detector. Unless it is otherwise clear, the discussion of this chapter (and, indeed, this whole book) will refer equally to Si(Li) and HPGe detectors. Very briefly, we shall also mention the recently introduced silicon drift detector, and an altogether different detector technology, the microcalorimeter.

3.2 The semiconductor X-ray detector

3.2.1 Principles of operation

Imagine that we have a perfect single crystal of a semiconductor, cooled, as described in the last chapter, so that leakage currents are negligible. If an X-ray photon of moderate energy (a few keV) enters the crystal, it will, in all probability, excite a photoelectron, which will have the energy of the photon, less the ionization energy. The photoelectron will travel through the crystal (typically, over less than 1 μm), exciting further electron–hole pairs as it goes. It is easy to see that this process will continue until all the electrons have a kinetic energy less than the band gap. Hence the average energy to produce an electron–hole pair will be between one and two times the band gap. In fact there are other ways that an electron can lose energy, without exciting further ionizations; the overall average energy per electron-hole pair in reality is therefore rather higher than our simple argument would predict. In Si, for example, the band gap is 1.1 eV, while it takes on average about 3.8 eV to excite each electron–hole pair. In Ge, the values are, respectively, 0.67 eV and 2.98 eV. Nevertheless, the end result is a cloud of electrons and holes, whose number is proportional to the energy of the incoming X-ray. If an electric field is maintained across the crystal, the electrons and holes will be attracted to opposite electrodes; the result will be the appearance of a charge at the electrode, proportional to the energy of the incoming X-ray. Although laborious to describe, this entire process takes place very fast, so the charge appears to come as a single pulse.

X-ray detectors may be constructed from a number of different materials, with different attributes. For electron microscopy applications, the choice almost always is either Si or Ge. Ge can be made pure enough to work well as a detector – hence the term 'high-purity' germanium or HPGe; Si, though, always has an excess of electron acceptors after purification. Hence, Li, an electron donor, is intentionally diffused into the Si in a carefully controlled way, to cancel out, or 'compensate', the excess acceptors, to give the material intrinsic, high resistivity properties. This process, of course, leads to the name 'lithium-drifted' Si, or Si(Li) detectors.

3.2.2 Structure of the detector

For practical reasons, the electrodes are made in the form of a very thin p-type region on one side, and an n-type region on the other, giving the device the structure of a p-i-n diode. When reverse-biased, the i-, or intrinsic, region can be made several millimetres thick. The p-layer is made with a very thin gold film deposited on the surface of the crystal. This face serves as the X-ray entrance window. The detector is very carefully designed to control the electric field – if electrons reach the edges, for example, they are trapped, and the resulting detected charge will be too small. For the same reason, it is essential that the crystal be perfectly clean, as any surface contamination can interfere with the shape of the electric field. Typical crystals used to detect X-rays in electron microscopy applications are from 1 to 3 mm thick, and have a surface area in the range 10–30 mm².

Even assuming we can collect the charge produced, the levels are very low; for a C X-ray at 284 eV, detected in a Si(Li) detector, we would see about 72 electrons, or a charge of 1.1×10^{-17} C. The amplifying circuit will not be discussed in detail here. However, it is essential that the total capacitance be kept low. As an example, although it does not represent exactly how the amplifier works, we can see that if the capacitance of the electrode and external circuit is about 5 pF (as is typical) the voltage change because of the charge would be less than 3 μV. This level of capacitance can only be attained through very careful design; typically a field-effect transistor (FET) chip (without can or leads) is directly connected to the rear electrode of the detector crystal. This amplifies the signal enough so that it can be brought out to a more conventional external amplifier.

3.2.3 Cooling the detector

As has been suggested above, it is necessary to cool the detector. A simple and effective method is to mount it, together with the pre-amplifier transistor, on the end of a Cu rod that is cooled by liquid nitrogen. Interestingly, the FET noise tends to go through a minimum at some temperature above that of liquid nitrogen; it is usual, therefore, to build-in an adjustable electric heater for the FET so the noise can be optimized, though this feature also adds to the circuit capacitance. Other designs, intended for situations when the supply of liquid nitrogen is inconvenient or unreliable, incorporate thermo-electric coolers, or small mechanical refrigerators. The former tend not to be able to reach low temperatures, and so suffer from poorer noise performance. The latter have the disadvantages of moving parts and fluids, potentially causing vibration problems with the microscope, and also greater complexity, leading to poorer reliability. Both are more expensive than a standard liquid nitrogen-cooled detector, and neither would be chosen unless the circumstances demanded it.

A consequence of the need to cool the detector is the need to protect it from the environment. Even in the vacuum of a modern electron microscope, a surface cooled to liquid nitrogen temperature will condense molecules from the atmosphere at the rate of about a monolayer per second, or roughly 10 nm h^{-1}. Most of these molecules will be water vapour, which will evaporate on warming the system, but some will be oil and other contaminants that will be difficult to remove, thus compromising the detector performance, as was described above. In any case, especially in SEMs, it is frequently necessary to vent the specimen chamber, to exchange samples or for other reasons. Hence the detector is built into its own clean vacuum system. The typical nitrogen-cooled system will make the liquid nitrogen do double-duty, serving also to cool a charge of molecular sieve which works as a sorption pump, capable of maintaining a vacuum in the 10^{-9} torr range for many years in a leak-free system. Even at this vacuum, though, in many detectors there is a sufficient leak rate that a layer of ice and other contaminants will slowly accumulate. This has consequences that we will discuss later in this chapter.

3.2.4 Detector windows

The difficulty of the closed vacuum system is that a way must be provided for X-rays to enter. One possibility is a mechanical valve (which might take the form of a rotatable 'turret'). This is very cumbersome, prone to leakage or accident, and quite an unsatisfactory solution in general. Nevertheless, for some special applications, valved detectors of one form or another were relatively popular in the 1980s, and a few are still in use today. For most purposes, though, the detector is built with some form of vacuum-tight 'window' of material that is relatively transparent to X-rays and yet is strong enough to withstand atmospheric pressure. For the first 20 years after the introduction of the Si(Li) EDX detector, the only practicable window was a thin foil of beryllium. Foils as thin as 7 μm could be made, capable of forming a window 10 mm^2 which could withstand atmospheric pressure. These windows would transmit most X-rays at energies above about 2 keV, but the transmission drops as the X-ray energy falls below

2 keV, and virtually all X-rays from the K-lines of the elements lighter than Na are absorbed. Unfortunately for the analyst, this inaccessible range includes a number of interesting elements. An unrelated disadvantage of the beryllium window is that the metal is toxic. Circumstances leading to the fracture of a window can release fine particles of beryllium metal or oxide, which can be inhaled – the worst form of ingestion. Much effort was expended, therefore, to develop alternative window materials which would still withstand the atmospheric pressure, and yet would transmit a useful fraction of the X-rays for elements as light as boron, and not have the toxicity of Be.

Starting in about 1988, such windows became commercially available, and today at least four general types are manufactured, including diamond, boron nitride, silicon nitride and various forms of polymer. *Table 3.1* (adapted from Lund, 1995) shows the transmission of X-rays from various light elements through typical thicknesses of these materials (the material designated AP1 is a polymer material marketed to detector manufacturers by Moxtek Corp). As can be seen, the polymer and nitride windows perform quite similarly, and transmit a good fraction of all the light element X-rays down to boron. All are reported to perform well in terms of durability. Different manufacturers offer different choices of window material for their detectors, but this need not be the determining factor when selecting a vendor – other differences between products will, except in a few cases, be more significant.

No thin window material is strong enough to be self-supporting against atmospheric pressure over the area of a detector crystal. Hence a support structure (typically of etched Si or tungsten wire) must be employed. This has the inevitable effect of blocking some of the X-rays. A well-designed support can have an open area of 80%, so the loss of signal is modest, though not insignificant. It is sometimes possible to see X-rays arising from fluorescence of the material of the grid.

Semiconductor X-ray detectors are sensitive to visible light, which is transmitted by the thin window materials. Many materials fluoresce in the visible or near-visible region under electron bombardment, and there can be other light sources in the microscope. It is therefore usual to coat the window with 40 nm of Al, which reflects most of the incident light, while

Table 3.1. Computed transmission of a variety of typical thin window structures for a selection of low-energy X-rays (adapted from Lund, 1995)

Window	Be K_α	B K_α	C K_α	N K_α	O K_α	F K_α	Na K_α
AP1	0.07	0.24	0.58	0.39	0.52	0.61	0.71
Polyimide	0.10	0.27	0.61	0.38	0.57	0.75	0.78
BN	0.09	0.26	0.20	0.36	0.42	0.58	0.74
Si_3N_4	0.00	0.01	0.15	0.43	0.41	0.61	0.90
Diamond	0.04	0.14	0.36	0.03	0.13	0.29	0.51

Note that in each case a 40-nm-thick coating of Al has been assumed.

absorbing only a small fraction of the X-rays (the window transmission data of *Table 3.1* incorporate the absorption in such an Al film). In addition, HPGe detectors, by virtue of their smaller band gap, are also sensitive to thermal IR radiation. For these detectors, it is necessary to incorporate a cooled Al foil between the detector and the vacuum window. This adds further absorption of the soft X-rays.

3.2.5 *Collimation of the detector*

X-rays can arise in the microscope not only from the point of intersection of the electron beam with the sample, but from almost any surface which is in the region of the specimen. To prevent these X-rays from reaching the detector, a physical collimator is fitted in front of the crystal. The collimator is made from a heavy material such as tantalum, and to prevent fluorescence of X-rays from the collimator, it is usually coated with a light material such as carbon dag. To get the most benefit from the collimator, it is usually designed with close tolerances, so even a small misalignment can seriously degrade the signal. When operating the microscope, it will be necessary to incorporate procedures to confirm the accuracy of the alignment and specimen position.

The detector, of course, can only intercept and measure those X-rays that reach it; it is an advantage, therefore, to position it as close to the sample as possible. However, this makes it difficult to design an effective collimator, especially in the TEM, in which, as we shall describe in Chapter 6, there is very limited space. For this, and other reasons, the design of the detector and collimator assembly is, to some extent, a compromise.

3.2.6 *Protection against spurious electron bombardment*

One of the products of the interaction of the electron beam with the sample is a flux of backscattered electrons, with energies up to that of the incident beam. These electrons are emitted essentially isotropically, and if allowed to enter the X-ray detector, can have a number of undesirable effects. At the least, the energy of each electron can be recorded as if it were an incoming X-ray, contributing a significant background to the spectrum. Worse, the electron, especially if of energies typical of TEMs, can inflict temporary or semi-permanent damage to the detector crystal by creating long-lived bulk or surface excited states which act directly as recombination centres or which degrade the field shape in the crystal. It is therefore necessary to prevent these electrons from reaching the detector, even at times when X-ray spectra are not being recorded.

The electrons lose some energy as they pass through the window. However, this is rarely enough protection. In SEM applications, it is usually adequate to install a small pair of permanent magnets between the collimator and the crystal. The field from these magnets deflects the backscattered electrons so that they do not strike the detector. This arrangement is called an 'electron trap', for obvious reasons, and is ubiquitously applied by manufacturers.

The case of the TEM is more complex. Firstly, the backscattered electrons have a much higher energy and require a higher field to deflect them (300 keV is common, and 400 keV and higher voltage microscopes are in use). Secondly, as we have mentioned, the detector must be placed as close as possible to the sample, actually between the pole-pieces of the objective lens of the microscope. In this position, an electron trap would both extend the distance from the detector to the sample, and the magnetic field of the trap would interfere severely with the field of the lens, creating image shift and astigmatism. However, because, in normal use, the magnetic field of the objective lens itself is extremely strong, the backscattered electrons tend to be confined to the magnetic lines of force, and are guided towards the lens pole-pieces. It has been found in practice that a detector placed at a relatively small take-off angle to the plane of the sample is not bombarded with a significant flux of electrons (this is not true for 'high take-off angle' detectors). Thus it is possible to perform excellent analysis without an electron trap. The difficulty arises when an excessive flux of backscatter electrons is produced, for example, during sample translation when the electron beam falls on a thick part of the sample or a gridbar, or when the objective lens must be turned off, either deliberately (for low-magnification operation, for example) or accidentally or incidentally. A number of solutions have been implemented to cope with these situations. None is entirely satisfactory. The simplest technique is to require that the detector be retracted from the sample, either manually (inexpensive but unreliable) or automatically. The automatic retraction can be triggered either by the act of switching the microscope to a non-protected mode, or by the detector electronics detecting an excessive signal. The main disadvantage of this method is the slow response time. An altogether better solution for most users is to incorporate a mechanical shutter, which can close automatically when the electronics detects an overload situation (suggesting the presence of electrons) or when the microscope is switched to an unsafe operating mode. The disadvantage with this approach is that the shutter assembly takes up space in front of the detector. As we have already mentioned, this space is precious, and can ill-afford to be lost. A compromise is an arrangement whereby the electron beam is blanked when the detector is overloaded. The detector can then be retracted before work proceeds. This arrangement is relatively safe for the detector, but involves a degree of interaction between the microscope and the detector electronics, which will probably require implementation by the user. In addition, some microscopes require that some specific aperture be in place for effective blanking – this may not be a convenient requirement for the operator. Despite all these difficulties, Si(Li) detectors have been used on TEMs (including dedicated scanning transmission instruments) for many years, and have given sterling service. It may be that they are more prone to performance degradation because of high-energy electron bombardment than those used on SEMs, but it is probably also true that detectors on SEMs are more prone to window damage due to accidents moving the stage, or, in the case of thin-window detectors, due to bombardment by particles of dust stirred up by the gas flow during venting of the chamber.

3.2.7 General mechanical details

It is convenient to build the X-ray detector as an integrated unit, independent of the microscope structure. It must therefore be built with a mechanical and vacuum interface to the microscope. Each microscope will be different, and will therefore have a different interface design. Generally, though, the interface will need to provide mechanical support for the liquid nitrogen container (cryostat) with its charge, and a means of adjusting the position of the detector crystal quite precisely in the microscope (in the TEM, it is common to require positioning tolerances of well under 1 mm). A vacuum seal will also be needed, of course. This latter function has usually been performed by a sliding 'O'-ring seal in the past, and indeed on many SEMs this continues to be adequate. For TEMs, though, a stainless bellows seal is far more satisfactory, the added cost being minor when compared to the improved vacuum cleanliness achieved. *Figure 3.1* is a schematic of a typical detector designed for 'line-of-sight' insertion, where the X-rays enter the detector parallel with the axis of the support tube. *Figure 3.2* shows a photograph of a typical SEM detector (in this case with a pneumatically operated shutter), on the bench, with the components indicated. *Figure 3.3* is a close-up photograph of the crystal and mount from the same detector, again with the components labelled, and *Figure 3.4* shows the collimator. *Figure 3.5* shows a typical TEM installation. An EDX system mounted on an electron microprobe, which would also be typical of an SEM installation, is shown later in this book in *Figure 8.1*.

It will be appreciated that many of the design features of EDX detectors involve compromises, and while 'standard' values of these compromises have evolved, it is still perfectly reasonable to order a detector made in

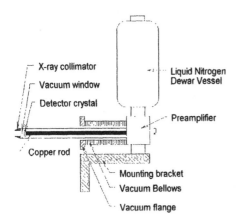

Figure 3.1. Sketch of the major components of a typical X-ray detector, in which the X-rays enter the detector parallel to the axis of the support tube.

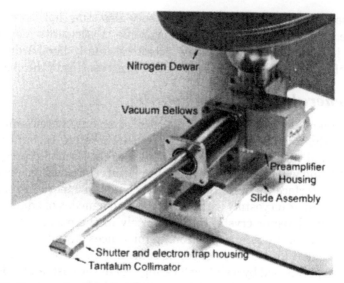

Figure 3.2. Photograph of a typical SEM detector (in this case, fitted with a pneumatically operated shutter). Certain components related to the mounting arrangements, have been removed.

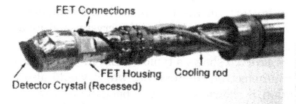

Figure 3.3. A close-up photograph of the detector components of the same detector as shown in *Figure 3.2*, with the outer tube and collimator removed.

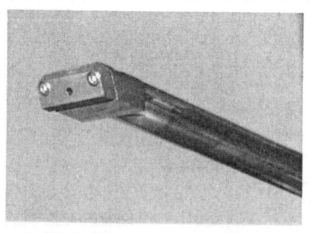

Figure 3.4. The collimator of the detector of *Figure 3.2*.

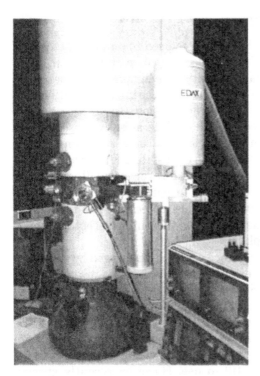

Figure 3.5. A typical detector mounted on a TEM/STEM (in this case, a Philips CM30).

some non-standard way for a special purpose. For example, for use in a microscope with ultra-high vacuum, where the ultimate sensitivity to light elements is required, a windowless detector may be provided; where light-emitting materials are being analysed extensively, a window with an extra-thick Al coat might be required, and so on. Some of these changes are relatively minor – an extra-thick Al layer, for example. An ultra-high-vacuum compatible windowless detector, though, would need a complete re-evaluation of all the materials used in the construction of the detector (because the outgassing rates of many common structural materials – Al, for example – are incompatible with ultra-high vacuum), as well as a possibly complex design of valves, bellows and slides to allow for isolation of the detector when the microscope column is vented.

3.3 The X-ray analyser

There is much more to be said about the operation of Si(Li) and HPGe detectors; we will get to that presently. We will first discuss the electronics and display systems into which the detector is interfaced.

3.3.1 The FET and detector reset

Earlier in this chapter we said that a FET is used to amplify the charge output of the detector crystal. We now need to look at this stage in more detail. *Figure 3.6* is the electrical schematic of a simple charge-sensitive amplifier, whose output voltage is proportional to the input charge. This, of course, is exactly what is required for the application. (In practice, a more complex feedback amplifier is used, but the considerations we discuss here are equally applicable.) What happens, though, as X-rays continue to arrive, and charge pulses accumulate at the gate of the FET? Obviously the output voltage cannot continue to increase forever – it will eventually saturate. One solution is to add a resistor in parallel with the feedback capacitor; this was in fact done in the earliest detectors. The main difficulty is the capacitance of the resistor, and its inherent noise, both of which limited the noise level of the amplifier.

It was soon found that the capacitance could be discharged by shining a pulse of light on the FET – this excites charge across the reverse-biased gate-source junction. This 'pulsed-optical' reset, as it is called, is triggered by a circuit that monitors the output voltage of the FET and pulses the LED when a predetermined value is reached. The output of the FET, therefore, is a step function, each step corresponding to the arrival of an X-ray, with, every so often, a sudden reset to the lower level. Many of these pulsed-optical reset systems are still in use. However, recently, special purpose-designed FETs have been introduced, incorporating special electrodes within the structure, allowing for controlled charge-injection resets, which are faster than pulsed-optical, and have other advantages too. Modern detectors from all manufacturers incorporate FETs of this type.

3.3.2 The pulse processor

The output from the FET is amplified at the detector by a pre-amplifier of relatively conventional design. The signal is then passed into a device known as a 'pulse processor'. At the time of writing, all-digital pulse processors are just coming onto the market. In these units, the pre-amplifier output is digitized at a high rate, the resulting digital data stream being subject to digital signal processing to extract and measure the pulses. The vast majority of the units in the field still operate with

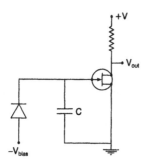

Figure 3.6. Electrical schematic of a simple charge-sensitive amplifier, whose output voltage is proportional to the input charge.

analogue or hybrid pulse processing, however. The digital pulse processors do essentially the same thing, but do it better, with added flexibility because of the software implementation of the required functions.

The pulse processor has the job of separating the signals from the noise, and presenting the pulses in an amplified and shaped form to an analogue-to-digital converter for digitization. The processor circuitry is by no means simple. Very fast pulses (the total charge collection time is typically a few tens of nanoseconds) must be extracted from significant noise, and quantified precisely. This must be done quickly, because the system must be ready to accept a new pulse as soon as possible, to avoid data loss. The basic idea is the same for all analogue systems, though there are a number of variations, some proprietary, which manufacturers will offer to suggest that their system is superior to those of competitors. There may indeed be some justification for these claims, but one can deduce that the differences are small, since no one design has become universal.

Principles In an analogue pulse processor, the principle is to divide the data stream in two. The first one is amplified by a short time-constant circuit, driving a discriminator. This senses when pulses exceeding some preset height are encountered, and turns on, or 'gates on' the other signal route. The signal in this case passes through a delay line, and then into an amplifier with a longer time constant. The variations from design to design have to do with the way that the gating of the signal is performed, and the way the amplifier time constant is set and changed. The ideal is an 'adaptive' time constant that can respond more slowly to small pulses (which are more affected by noise), or when a longer period is available after a pulse arrives before the next one is encountered, and reset the system quickly to be ready to deal with the next pulse. It is these functions that can more easily be implemented in software than in hardware.

Time constant While in digital pulse processors an appropriate time constant is always selected automatically, in analogue processors a base time constant must be preset. This was done in older systems with a front-panel switch, and in more recent ones by software. The selection of time constant is important because it determines the compromise that is made between the maximum data collection rate and the resolution with which the X-rays are identified. We shall discuss both these properties in detail later. The difficulty of changing time constants is that inevitably there are small associated changes in amplifier gain; these manifest themselves as changes in calibration of the X-ray spectrum. In the fully analogue systems, the gain and zero calibration were set by potentiometers on the front panel; a change in time constant therefore required a manual recalibration of the gain. The user was therefore strongly discouraged, as a practical matter, from making frequent changes in the time constant. As we shall see, this makes it harder to select optimum operating conditions for all the things one might want to do during an analysis session. The great advantage of the digitally controlled pulse processors is that appropriate gain and zero values can be predetermined and stored for each time constant. Selecting a new time constant can therefore cause the appropriate calibration to be loaded automatically. The user can change time constants at any time during an experiment with a few clicks of the mouse (or equivalent) and continue working essentially without interruption.

Strobed zero peak and system performance Some pulse processors incorporate a design feature whereby a free-running oscillator periodically gates on (or 'strobes') the measurement channel when an X-ray has not been detected. The resulting signal should indicate the arrival of a 'pulse' of zero energy, and is used by the system as a way of setting the system zero dynamically, rather than relying on preset values. Displaying this signal on the monitor provides the operator with a convenient way of assessing the system performance, as the 'resolution' of the resulting 'peak' on the display directly relates to the noise in the system. Degraded noise performance can arise from degraded components, bad connections, microphony from mechanical interference, direct electrical interference, ground loops and any number of other problems. It should be part of the normal practice of the operator to monitor the performance of the system, whether by monitoring this 'strobed zero' peak (when available) or by acquiring spectra of standard samples in known conditions. In fact many modern software packages incorporate routines that indicate the 'system' resolution. While the definition of 'system' in this usage may differ from manufacturer to manufacturer, consistent use of these routines will certainly monitor whether any changes are taking place in the performance.

3.3.3 Multi-channel analyser

The rest of the electronic chain is relatively unimportant as far as determining the quality of spectra is concerned (though differences from manufacturer to manufacturer, or even system to system, may make a very big difference as to how convenient or otherwise a system is to use for a particular purpose). The analogue-to-digital conversion is quite straightforward. A computer reads the digital value giving the energy of the photon, and increments the number in the memory location corresponding to that energy. Typical energy bands, or channels, are 10 or 20 eV wide, though for special purposes other widths may be selected. The computer then displays the spectrum as a histogram of counts versus channel (or energy). *Figure 3.7* is an example of a typical spectrum, showing the energy range from zero to 18 keV, while *Figure 3.8* shows the Fe K_α peak expanded so the individual channels of the histogram are visible. This spectrum is from a low-alloy steel analysed in a transmission instrument operating at 250 kV, and illustrates a number of features which are identified on the plot and in the caption, which we will describe in later paragraphs.

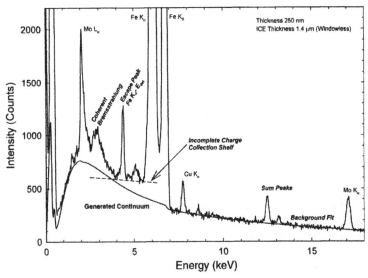

Figure 3.7. Typical EDX spectrum, in this case of a low-alloy steel obtained in a TEM. Characteristic and bremsstrahlung continuum X-rays are indicated, as are sum, escape and coherent bremsstrahlung peaks. In addition, some contribution of degraded events (indicated as the Incomplete Charge Collection Shelf) is visible. The generated continuum is a purely theoretical background shape, normalized in intensity to the measured spectrum in the region labelled 'Background Fit'.

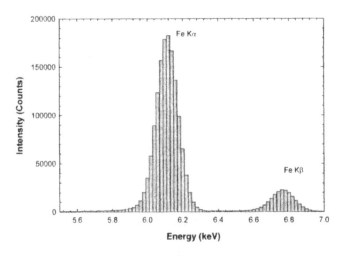

Figure 3.8. The region of the Fe K-peak of *Figure 3.7*, plotted on a very different scale, making the individual channels of the spectrum histogram obvious.

3.4 Details of the spectrum

How information is extracted from the spectrum and interpreted will be the subject of later chapters in this book. Before we proceed, though, we must examine some more of the features of an X-ray spectrum as recorded from a semiconductor detector, as we will need this information in order to be able to interpret these spectra.

3.4.1 Characteristic peaks

The most prominent features of the spectrum in *Figure 3.7* are the 'peaks', corresponding to the energies of the characteristic X-rays, which we described in the preceding chapter. These peaks, though, are not one channel wide, but spread over a number of adjacent channels. Critical examination of the spectrum will reveal that the width of the peaks is actually a function of the energy. The fact that the X-rays are not recorded at one specific energy has important consequences for the analyst, as we shall see in later chapters of this book. For now we will simply discuss why this happens.

Energy resolution Thinking back to how the charge pulse is produced in the detector, we recall that the average number of electron–hole pairs produced in the crystal by a particular incident X-ray is given by the energy of the X-ray divided by the average energy required to create a single electron–hole pair. It is clear that there will be some variation from X-ray to X-ray of the total charge produced. We might try to calculate this on the basis of a simple statistical argument, which might predict that, when measuring X-rays of energy E, the distribution would be Gaussian with a centroid

$$n = \frac{E}{\varepsilon} \tag{3.1}$$

and a variance

$$\sigma = \sqrt{n} \tag{3.2}$$

where ε is the mean energy to create an electron–hole pair. However, a careful consideration will show that the simple statistical argument is invalid in this case, as it describes a data collection situation that is different from ours. In particular we have the constraint that the total energy given up must be that of the X-ray for each event, not simply an average over all events. In fact, it is found that while the peak is Gaussian, and the centroid is given by Equation 3.1, the variance is actually

$$\sigma = \sqrt{Fn} \tag{3.3}$$

where F is called the Fano factor, and has the value of about 0.11–0.12 for a Si(Li) detector, and about 0.13 for a HPGe detector. (Confusingly, an alternative, but mathematically equivalent definition of the Fano factor, with a different numerical value, is also in use. Our description is from Lowe, the alternative can be found, for example, in Woldseth.) We can work through the numbers, and calculate that for a Si(Li) detector the resolution at 5.9 keV (the Mn K_α energy – conventionally used as a reference energy for detectors) would be expected to be of the order of 120 eV. The equivalent number for HPGe would be about 113 eV. For an O X-ray at 532 eV we would expect a resolution of about 35 eV for Si(Li) and about 34 eV for HPGe.

Electronic noise These estimates are, of course, lower bounds on the achievable resolution; other issues, such as electronic noise, will degrade the actual resolution. There are a number of contributions to electronic noise, of which the most significant for the detection and measurement of X-rays in the semiconductor detector is called series noise, which depends strongly upon the capacitance at the gate of the FET. In fact, improvement in FET technology, mainly in reducing the effective gate capacitance, is arguably the largest single contributor to the improvement in detector resolution over the last 20 years. Be that as it may, series noise decreases as the time constant of the measuring circuit increases. Hence a way to decrease the noise and improve the resolution is to increase the time constant. This is illustrated in *Figure 3.9*, where we show, overlaid, spectra from a stainless steel acquired at time constants of 4 and 100 μs, respectively. The spectra were acquired for the same livetime (a measurement which we shall discuss later), and the peaks contain essentially the same number of counts. The change in resolution is clear, especially in the lower energy region.

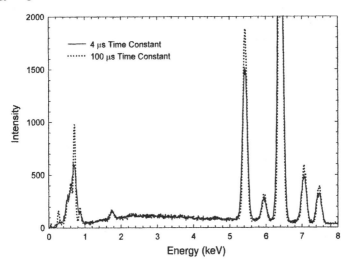

Figure 3.9. Overlay of measured SEM spectra from a stainless steel, obtained at processor time constants of 4 and 100 μs, with the same number of counts in each spectrum, illustrating how the longer time constant leads to narrower and taller spectral peaks.

Theoretical considerations suggest that with present-day technology, for a 10 mm^2 detector the lower limit of electronic noise is about 50 eV at a time constant of about 40 μs for a Si(Li) detector. If the noise sources are independent, they add in quadrature; that is:

$$N^2 = n_1{}^2 + n_2{}^2 \tag{3.4}$$

where N represents the total noise, and n_1 and n_2 are the independent sources. This is plotted in *Figure 3.10* for both a theoretical Si(Li) detector and a HPGe detector operated in optimum conditions as a function of energy, from zero to 20 keV. As the capacitance of the detector varies with the area, a larger detector would have somewhat poorer resolution. Likewise, the dielectric constant of Ge is higher than that of Si, so HPGe detectors have higher capacitance, and hence electronic noise, than Si(Li) detectors of the same area, partially offsetting the anticipated advantage of the improved statistics because of the reduced energy per electron-hole pair of the HPGe detector. The HPGe detector gains, though, because, for a given X-ray pulse, the output charge pulse is larger, so the signal-to-noise ratio in the electronics is better, and an HPGe detector is expected to have lower noise throughout the spectrum, as shown in the figure.

Modern premium Si(Li) detectors from all manufacturers actually fall very close to this curve, at least when operated at low count rates. There is thus little reason to hope for significant improvement in the resolution of these detectors in the future. This is the main reason for the interest in HPGe detectors. Modern HPGe detectors tend to outperform the Si(Li) detectors as far as resolution is concerned, but not by as much as would be expected from these considerations, because of other difficulties that will be discussed later.

We note that digital pulse processing does not change the preceding argument – the advantages of digital pulse processing do not include better ultimate resolution, but they do include improved signal throughput at a given resolution – the topic of the next section.

Livetime and dead time We can think of adding a time constant to a measurement circuit as simply taking longer to make the measurement, averaging the noise and therefore arriving at a more precise final value.

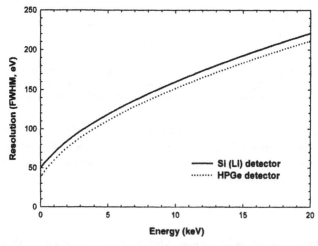

Figure 3.10. Theoretical limit of the resolution of Si(Li) and HPGe detectors, as a function of X-ray energy.

The difficulty is, of course, that the longer it takes to make a single measurement, the fewer measurements can be made in total. As we shall see later in this book, the total number of counts acquired is at least as important as the resolution of the spectrum. An associated problem is that of dealing with overlapping X-rays – when a second X-ray arrives at the detector before the first is fully processed.

Different manufacturers use slightly different techniques, at least in analogue pulse processors, to minimize the time from when an X-ray arrives until the detector is ready to accept the next one, and we need not be concerned with the details of how this is done. In fact there are two problems. If two X-rays arrive so close together in time that the second would interfere with the processing of the first, both must be discarded. This case is dealt with by a coincidence detector, which aborts the slow-channel processing which was triggered for the first X-ray. No count is recorded, although it is still necessary to wait for the slow channel to recover before another X-ray can be accepted. In the second case, the second X-ray arrives after the signal from the first has been passed to the slow channel. In this case, processing of the first X-ray can continue, the second only being discarded. This is dealt with by a signal internal to the processor which indicates when the slow channel is busy, and which, when active, prevents another pulse from being gated into the slow channel. Even though the second pulse is not fully processed, it is still necessary to wait some time for the amplifier to settle before another pulse can be accepted. This time may or may not extend the time the processor is busy processing the first X-ray. The busy signal would, of course, also be asserted by the overlap described above when both signals are discarded. The time during which the detector is busy is called 'dead time'.

It can be clearly seen that as the rate of arrival of X-rays at the detector increases, the fraction that are not measured increases. It is not quite so obvious, but clear after a moment's reflection, that after some critical count rate, the rate of detection actually falls as the arrival rate increases (this argument makes the reasonable assumption that the X-ray generation is stochastic). *Figure 3.11* shows a plot of a simulation of this effect.

All commercial pulse processor and analyser combinations incorporate a measurement of 'livetime'. Simply put, this is the time during which the system is not busy, and therefore is capable of recording the arrival of an incoming X-ray. Almost always, the operator selects a desired amount of livetime for the spectral acquisition, rather than real time (i.e. time as would be measured on a stopwatch). For many applications of EDX analysis, the livetime, or the indication of the dead time, is a convenience to the operator, showing quickly when the X-ray arrival rate is inappropriate. However, for quantitative analysis in the SEM, an accurate knowledge of the rate of production of the X-rays may be required. In this case, a reliable livetime indicator is essential to the performance of the analysis.

It is possible to blank the electron beam very fast (in less than 1 μs). This raises the possibility of blanking the beam as soon as an X-ray is detected, thus minimizing the chance of a second X-ray arriving and spoiling the

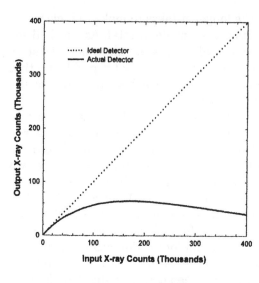

Figure 3.11. Simulation of the number of X-rays detected (in 10 s) as a function of the number arriving at the detector, for an amplifier time constant of 10μs.

measurement. When the detector and pulse processor are ready to process another X-ray, the beam can be unblanked again. Such arrangements have been implemented and do work. It can be shown that in terms of the real time conducting the experiment, this system can result in up to a fourfold increase in the rate of collection of X-rays. However, to achieve this collection rate, the electron beam must, usually, be extremely large. Often, this will not be an acceptable condition. However, the implementation is relatively easy, and the gain in count rate is certainly worthwhile if the experimental details permit it to be achieved.

3.4.2 *Spurious responses in the system*

In this chapter we shall discuss only those spurious responses that are inherent in the detector operation. Discussion of the detection of real X-rays, which are 'spurious' only insofar as they do not arise as a primary result of the interaction of the electron beam with the sample, will be delayed until later chapters.

Pulse pile-up Although the pile-up rejection circuit, as it is known, has good performance, it is still possible for two X-rays to arrive at the detector at so nearly the same time that the electronics fails to recognize that there are two pulses. In this case, the charge from both will be summed by the pulse processor, and the event will be recorded as a single X-ray whose energy is the sum of the energies of the two actual X-rays. If enough of these events take place, a spurious peak will appear in the spectrum, known, obviously, as a 'sum' peak. The intensity of the sum peak with respect to the parent is a function of the count rate. Thus a suspected sum peak in a spectrum may be confirmed by recording a new spectrum at significantly lower count rate. A real peak will not change in relative intensity; a sum peak will be reduced. In general the most significant sum peak will usually correspond to two X-rays from the major peak, but as pile-up rejection is generally less efficient for X-rays of lower energy, a moderately intense low-energy peak may generate a larger sum peak than a more intense peak of higher energy. *Figure 3.7* shows some examples of sum peaks. If the pulse pile-up rejection is not working properly (or in very old systems with early designs of pile-up rejection) more complex pile-up 'shelves' may be observed, but modern designs have effectively eliminated these. See an older textbook (for example, Woldseth) for more information about these effects.

Digital processing of the pulses can significantly improve throughput at given resolution, and reduce the size of sum peaks. It can do nothing, though, for the spurious responses we discuss next, and which originate in the detector crystal itself.

Escape peaks In the discussion in Chapter 2 on the production of electron–hole pairs within the detector crystal, we greatly simplified the processes at work. Before the final generation of the electron–hole pairs, all sorts of other excitations can take place. One will usually be the ionization of a core-level electron of the detector crystal, leaving behind a vacancy, which is subsequently filled with the emission of a characteristic X-ray. Indeed, this is the very same process that generates the X-rays that are being analysed, except that the initial ionization is caused in the sample by electron bombardment rather than by X-ray excitation. The X-ray propagates through the crystal, and usually will be reabsorbed, creating a new photoelectron and subsequent chain of electron–hole pairs, which all contribute to the final pulse of charge. All is, therefore, well, and the energy of the incident X-ray is determined correctly. However, the characteristic X-ray stands a non-negligible chance of reaching the surface of the crystal (or some other inactive region), in which case the energy it carries is lost. The analyser detects a pulse whose energy is equal to the energy of the incoming X-ray less the energy of the characteristic X-ray from the detector. In the case of Si, the only X-ray of significance is the K_α X-ray, with an energy of 1.74 keV. Hence spurious peaks can be generated at this energy below the parent peak in the spectrum. Examples are identified in *Figure 3.7*. It might be imagined that the escape peak would be more intense for incident X-rays that are absorbed close to the detector surface, and so it proves. In a Si(Li) detector, the escape peaks are observed to be most intense, as a fraction of the parent peak, for P X-rays, which are the most strongly absorbed by Si (and hence absorbed closest to the surface). *Table 3.2* presents the mean absorption depth in Si for X-rays from a selection of elements of common interest. (The data in this table for elements lighter than P is for later reference.) Fortunately for the analyst, a good semi-theoretical, semi-empirical model exists for the generation of escape peaks in a Si(Li) detector, and all commercial X-ray analysis systems incorporate routines, which work well, to process the spectrum and restore the counts in the escape peaks to the parent peaks.

Table 3.2. Mean absorption depth in Si for X-rays from a selection of elements of common interest

Element	Kα energy (keV)	Characteristic depth (μm)
C	0.277	0.12
N	0.392	0.27
O	0.525	0.53
Na	1.04	3.0
Mg	1.25	5.0
Al	1.49	8.0
Si	1.74	12.3
P	2.02	1.6
S	2.31	2.2
Ca	3.69	7.4
Ti	4.51	13
Cr	5.41	21
Fe	6.40	34

Unfortunately, the same is not true for HPGe detectors, and good escape peak correction remains, at least at the time of writing, an unreached goal for users of these systems. Fortune is on the side of the user, though, for the major escape energy is that of the Ge K_α line at 9.9 keV (the L escape at about 1.2 keV is not significant). X-ray peaks whose energy is below the Ge K excitation energy (11.1 keV) cannot, therefore, generate escape peaks. Many investigations are performed by analysis of X-rays in this energy range, especially in SEMs. Even if higher-energy X-rays are being detected, they tend (because of their energy) to penetrate further into the crystal before exciting a photoelectron. The resulting fluoresced X-ray therefore has to travel further through the crystal, and as a result is less likely to escape.

Compton scattering Another inherent interaction between the detector and the incident X-ray that can generate a spurious response, but this time not a peak, is Compton scattering. This is almost never seen in EDX spectra recorded on an SEM, and even on an intermediate-voltage TEM generates only a slight distortion of the background shape at low energies in the spectrum. It is nevertheless mentioned here for completeness, as effects due to Compton scattering can be seen in X-ray fluorescence experiments.

Compton scattering is an inelastic interaction between the incident X-ray and electrons in the solid, in which energy is transferred from the X-ray to the electrons. Provided the scattered X-ray goes on to be absorbed in a photoelectric event, all will be well, for the total energy will eventually be converted to charge that will be detected. The problem arises when the Compton-scattered X-ray escapes from the crystal. In this case a small amount of energy will be left behind and duly detected by the system and recorded as an X-ray of low energy. However, for X-rays below 20 keV the relative probability of Compton scattering, compared to photoelectric absorption, is low, and the probability of a Compton-scattered X-ray (which is typically deviated only a small amount from the initial path) escaping from the detector is almost zero, which is why Compton events are not seen in the SEM. Even if a Compton event is recorded, it will be at a very low energy (below 100 eV) as the total Compton energy change cannot exceed this value for incident X-rays below about 5 keV. In the intermediate-voltage TEM, X-rays of far higher energy are generated in the sample (though they may not be recorded in the spectrum). The probability of Compton scattering increases with X-ray energy until it is about equal to that for photoelectric absorption at about 50 keV for Si. However, the total probability of absorption in a typical Si(Li) detector is only about 20% for these X-rays, and the generation of X-rays of these energies is not very efficient, so the total number of Compton events recorded will still be small.

HPGe detectors are less prone to generate Compton events because the relative probability of Compton scattering to photoelectric absorption is far lower in this material than in Si.

Coherent bremsstrahlung A final source of peak-like features, seen only in TEMs, and then only in some samples, is coherent bremsstrahlung. These have nothing to do with the characteristic peaks in the X-ray spectrum itself, but arise from an interaction between the incident electrons and the periodic potential in crystalline samples, the details of which are complex. The position of the peaks varies both with the incident electron energy and the sample tilt, but not in a consistent way with sample chemistry. The peaks are typically observed in the energy range 2–10 keV, and there may be more than one order visible, higher orders being seen at multiples of the base energy. The width of coherent bremsstrahlung peaks is typically greater than that of characteristic peaks, though this depends upon details of the measurements. The intensity of the peaks is very low, typically appearing like a trace element at the level of 0.1% or so. In *Figure 3.7*, a first-order coherent bremsstrahlung peak is identified in the spectrum. The second-order peak would not be visible, even if it is present, because it is obscured by the low-energy tail of the main Fe K_α peak.

Incomplete charge collection and detector dead layer Another response, which may be termed 'spurious' in that it causes X-rays to be recorded at energies other than the correct one, is called generically 'incomplete charge collection'. (Some writers use the term 'degraded events' for this phenomenon.) As the name suggests, the problem arises when not all the charge from the electron–hole pairs reaches the electrodes, and the X-ray is recorded at some lower energy, which could be any value between zero and the energy of the parent peak. Incomplete charge collection can arise because of imperfections in the crystal, and as crystal manufacturing has improved, incomplete charge collection performance has improved. It can also arise, though, through surface contamination or short- or long-lived states within the crystal generated by energetic electron bombardment. A detector exhibiting bad incomplete charge collection can often be partially restored by a careful warm-up and pumping (but see the discussion later about warming detectors). It has been the authors' experience, however, that *in-house* efforts can never fully restore such a detector – usually at least a thorough cleaning of the crystal is required, if not replacement, by the vendor or other qualified contractor.

Another way that incomplete charge collection can arise is by the incoming X-ray being absorbed so close to the crystal surface (usually the entrance surface) that the electrons and/or holes reach the electrodes before all their energy has been converted to electron–hole pairs. In the extreme, the X-ray can be absorbed within the p-type electrode where the electric field is low, so the electrons are not accelerated away and have time to recombine. The charge is therefore totally lost. Because of this, the p-type electrode is often called the 'dead layer', and while there has been discussion about the appropriateness of this term, we will use it here. Manufacturers have worked hard to improve detectors to reduce the thickness of the dead layer, especially because it affects detection of the very light elements particularly severely (because the soft X-rays are absorbed closer to the crystal surface, as shown in *Table 3.2*). Modern Si(Li) detectors, when working properly, show very little incomplete charge collection. The same is not yet true of HPGe detectors, though. Partly this is because the X-rays are absorbed closer to the crystal surface (especially those from the light elements), and partly because manufacturers have not yet gained the many years of experience in production of these devices that they have in making Si(Li) crystals, so the details of the finish are not as perfect. Thus although a HPGe detector may have better resolution in terms of full width at half maximum (FWHM) of the peaks than a Si(Li) detector, in terms of peak/background performance at low energies (where the improved resolution is particularly desired) the Si(Li) may still perform better. This situation may be expected to change, though, as manufacturing technology for the HPGe detectors matures.

The degraded events identified in *Figure 3.7* represent a moderate manifestation of the phenomenon.

3.4.3 Detector icing

Earlier in this chapter we mentioned the possibility of ice condensing on the surfaces of the detector crystal. There are two consequences of this. The first is that X-rays have to pass through the ice layer before they reach the crystal, and can be absorbed in the process. This can severely degrade the low-energy sensitivity of a detector. Experience has shown that it is easily possible to get a layer of ice 1 μm thick or more on the crystal. *Figure 3.12* is a simulation of a spectrum of a nickel oxide film acquired by a windowless detector, with and without such a layer of ice. The effect is obvious. The second consequence of the ice is disturbance to the surfaces of the crystal, and the possible interference with the charge collection, as has

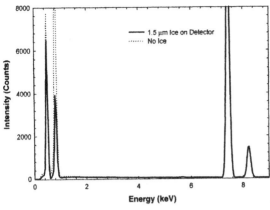

Figure 3.12. Simulation of spectra from a nickel oxide thin film in a TEM, acquired with a windowless detector with and without a layer of ice.

been mentioned. Since ice build-up occurs on virtually all liquid nitrogen-cooled detectors (the only difference being the rate, which depends upon the absence or presence of microleaks in the window or other structures of the detector, the choice of detector materials, how well they were degassed before assembly, the efficiency of the cryopumping agent and so on), it is essential, if performance is to be maintained, that provision is made to remove it. Several manufacturers make detectors that are intended to be warmed up, one (in a patent-protected arrangement) building in an integral heater to allow the crystal to warm up enough to sublime the ice without the need to drain the cryostat of its nitrogen. At least one other manufacturer has responded by building ultra-high vacuum detectors in which it is anticipated that the ice build-up will occur so slowly as to not be a nuisance. Time will tell if they are right.

Warming detectors Twenty years ago it was the general opinion that Si(Li) X-ray detectors should never be warmed up. Partly this arose from the misguided belief that the Li would drift out of the crystal (to be fair, if the detector was left warm for a prolonged period with the bias turned on, the Li could diffuse, but if the detector is warmed while switched on, it is likely that the FET will blow, too), partly it was because of a fear, certainly grounded in experience, that repeated cooling and warming cycles could cause mechanical problems because of differential thermal contraction, and partly in the observation that frequently after a heating/cooling cycle a detector would not quite regain its resolution specification. This last observation is probably explained as follows: during the warm-up the gas trapped in the molecular sieve is released (herein lies yet another problem – there can be so much gas that the detector becomes pressurized, and the window, being only designed to withstand atmospheric pressure from the outside, can then blow out). On subsequent re-cooling the vacuum does not fully recover before the crystal cools down. Therefore an ice layer re-condenses on the crystal, causing the incomplete charge collection problems we have already discussed, which degrade the resolution of the spectrum. The solution is to pump the detector when it is warm. This will require access to a pumping adapter for the pumping port, and a suitable vacuum system capable of reaching 10^{-6} mbar or below. While it is never a good idea to attempt home remedies such as this on detectors that are under warranty, or are otherwise in front-line service, new life has been breathed into many older systems by a careful warm-up and pump cycle. It is very important to stress the need for care when warming beryllium-windowed detectors, because of the toxicity of that material, and the health risks associated with fracturing the window. Perhaps the most important precaution to take is to establish the pumping before allowing the molecular sieve to warm up. In this way, even if the sieve is saturated, the pressure will not rise dangerously, and will always be negative in the detector volume. It might be observed at this point that while the complexity of a windowless detector brings many associated problems with the operation, these detectors are by far the easiest to warm up – you simply let the microscope vacuum system pump the detector (making sure, of course, that the pumping mode is appropriate for the anticipated gas load).

It is not intended that these comments serve as directions for warming a detector. The intention is to suggest that warming a 'dead' or 'moribund' system does, in fact, have a good chance of bringing it back to life. The user thinking of performing such a job should seek further advice, either from the detector manufacturer or from a knowledgeable colleague.

3.5 New detector technologies

Virtually all EDXS systems in use today use the technology that we have been describing in this chapter. It is likely that this situation will not change markedly at least for the next few years. There are, though, alternative EDX technologies, and we will conclude this chapter by discussing two of these briefly.

3.5.1 Silicon drift detector

The more well-developed detector is the silicon drift detector (SDD). The basic physical principle of operation of this detector is exactly the same as the standard detector we have been discussing. The difference is in the structure of the detector crystal itself. Instead of a very carefully maintained uniform electric field generated by the front and back electrodes, the SDD has a series of concentric electrodes designed to generate a controlled field shape in the crystal, steering the charge towards a very small collector electrode in the centre. Because the collector electrode is very small, its capacitance is far lower than that of the standard detector, which means that the system noise is much lower, and the amplifier time constant can be reduced. In turn, this means that the detector is capable of much higher count rates than the standard detectors. It also means that the detector need not be run at such low temperatures. In fact, good performance is achieved with only a simple thermo-electric cooling system, eliminating the need for liquid nitrogen. Detectors using this technology are commercially available.

There are, though, good reasons why, at least at the time of writing, these detectors are only used in a few cases. SDD technology is under very active research by manufacturers, and it is likely that what we write here will soon be out of date. However, at least at present, workable SDDs are smaller, both in active area and in thickness, than conventional crystals. They are also not yet capable of achieving such good energy resolution. We will come back to this in later chapters; suffice it for now to say that these disadvantages make the SDD unattractive except for a few specialized applications.

3.5.2 Microcalorimeter

The microcalorimeter detector uses an altogether different principle to measure the energy of incoming X-rays. The active element is a small piece of superconductor held at a temperature very close to the superconducting transition temperature. Absorption of an X-ray leads to a small and brief, but nevertheless quantifiable, decrease in the conductivity. The statistical precision of the measurement is far higher than the precision of detecting electron–hole pairs in the silicon detector, so the inherent energy resolution is much better. For low-energy peaks in a spectrum, it is capable of resolution comparable with that of a crystal spectrometer.

The interest in the microcalorimeter detector arises from attempts to improve the limited spatial resolution of X-ray analysis using conventional methods in the SEM; we will discuss the application more in that section of the book. Initial experiments have been performed to demonstrate that the concept does work, but much work remains to be done before systems can be built commercially. Compromises must be made in designing the sensor: for example, the need for low thermal capacity (to maximize the temperature rise for a small input of energy) means that the size must be small; therefore it collects only a few X-rays. However, if a more energetic X-ray is absorbed, the detector can saturate (completely losing its superconducting nature for a relatively prolonged time) because of the excessive temperature rise. Early systems will undoubtedly be dedicated to specialized applications. One area of research is in the use of focusing systems for the X-rays, to increase the collection efficiency. It will take at least this, or some other yet unforeseen, development in the technology before microcalorimeter detectors can be expected to be in general use.

4 Spectral processing

4.1 Introduction

It is time to look more closely at spectra, and discuss ways in which they may be processed to yield the numbers of counts required for analysis. For now, we will assume that we are interested only in the intensities of the characteristic peaks; we will discuss later the information that we may glean from the bremsstrahlung. We should mention that measuring major peaks, free of overlap, is, as we shall see, not particularly challenging. Even the simplest peak integral, obtained by defining a 'window' in the spectrum corresponding to those channels that contain a significant number of counts from the peak of interest, is surprisingly useful. The difficulties arise when trying to quantify the presence of a trace element, or measuring the concentration of elements whose spectral peaks overlap.

In this chapter we will discuss issues common to experiments in all forms of electron microscopes. Characteristics specific to either SEM or TEM analysis will be described in the respective chapters later in the book.

4.2 Background stripping

4.2.1 Window integrals

The first method is to set the window so that the channels at either extreme are at the level of the background. Then interpolate between these channels and subtract – a trivial task for a computer. This is illustrated in *Figure 4.1*. In a spectrum with good statistics (i.e. many counts), and for peaks that do not overlap each other, this works quite well. There are a number of problems, though. For example, the statistics of the background subtraction are limited by the numbers of counts in the two sampling channels (the two extreme channels). The user's choice of channels is also critical – especially for trace elements where the peak is only a little above the background. The required window width will vary with the resolution of the system, which is a function of the count rate and the system time constant (which can be changed by the user), and of the

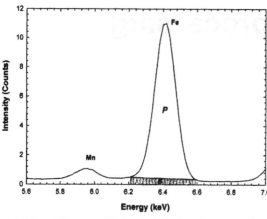

Figure 4.1. EDX spectrum of a steel sample, showing the peak and background regions prior to stripping.

energy of the X-ray line. If the detector is prone to incomplete charge-collection effects, the necessary window could be unreasonably (and unpredictably) large. All of these problems are illustrated schematically in *Figure 4.2*.

4.2.2 Polynomial curve fitting

Performing a polynomial fit to windows defined in background regions of the sample addresses several of the problems of the simple windowing technique. It does require user selection of the background windows, which must be selected to avoid not only minor characteristic peaks, but also spurious peaks such as sum, escape and coherent bremsstrahlung peaks. Older systems relied on this technique extensively, and it is still in use in current software, especially for SEM. It has two principal draw-backs: it is hard to model the background in the lower-energy region of the spectrum (because of the prevalence of spurious peaks and incomplete charge collection, and because absorption in thicker samples, or the detector windows, causes the background to vary rapidly in this region), and it does not take into account relatively sharp changes in the back-ground caused by absorption edges of major elements in a thicker sample. The method, and the drawbacks, are illustrated in *Figure 4.3*.

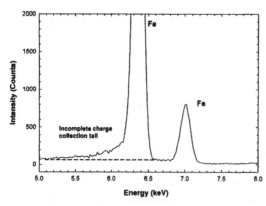

Figure 4.2. Similar to *Figure 4.1*, but with peak distortion due to degraded events, illustrating the difficulty of choosing an appropriate window for peak and background determination.

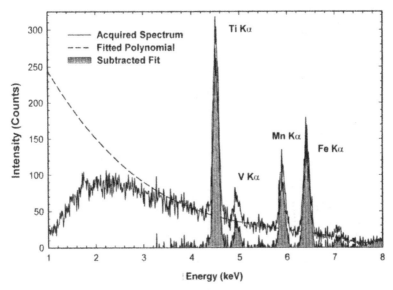

Figure 4.3. A spectrum from a Ti alloy, obtained in an SEM, with a background modelled by polynomial curve-fitting. For the purposes of this illustration, the fit to the spectrum at low energies has not been optimized. In practice, a better, though still usually poor, fit can be obtained.

4.2.3 Top-hat filtering

A popular semi-automatic method of removing the effects of the background is to use what is known as a 'top-hat' filter. This is a channel-by-channel convolution of the spectrum with a filter function. Space precludes a detailed description, but with an appropriately designed filter, the effect is to remove the slowly varying background and leave the rapidly changing peaks. Unfortunately the peaks are converted from their simple Gaussian form to a bipolar form unsuitable for direct extraction of a number of counts, but computer fitting of library spectra or theoretically generated peaks easily overcomes this problem. The method also has the benefit of adding a significant degree of smoothing to the spectrum. A minor drawback is that the ideal width of the filter function is itself a function of the energy resolution of the spectrum, which is, of course, variable. Therefore, the choice of the actual width is a compromise. This method is certainly more automatic, and less prone to user error than the polynomial fit method described above. However, it requires either a library spectrum of each element in the sample, or a reliable way of modelling the spectrum. Neither of these is necessarily easy to obtain. *Figure 4.4* shows a typical spectrum, and the result of performing top-hat filtering on it.

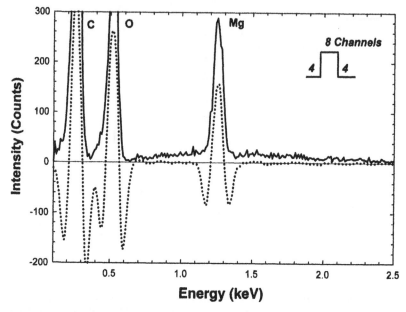

Figure 4.4. An example of background removal by top-hat filtering.

4.3 Background modelling

The main objection to all these background 'stripping' techniques is that the bremsstrahlung actually carries information about the sample. Not only that, but, compared with the characteristic peaks, there are relatively few counts in each background channel. Thus a background stripping technique that depends on only a few background channels is relatively imprecise because of the large statistical uncertainty. While this is not a major problem for the analysis of major peaks, it is a significant difficulty in the quantitative analysis of minor constituents. We have already mentioned the problem in the extreme case of using a single channel either side of the peak window to determine the correction. If, however, a reliable model of the background shape is available, the possibility arises of normalizing the model to a large number of channels (and hence a large number of counts) representing the background in the spectrum. It is also possible to select a region of the spectrum free of coherent bremsstrahlung, incomplete charge collection and other artifacts. The precision of the background subtraction can be significantly improved in this way.

Fortunately, as we mentioned in Chapter 2, such models have been derived. These can readily be incorporated into the analysis software package, taking account of absorption and fluorescence effects (which will be discussed in detail in the following two chapters). One such software package freely available is Desktop Spectrum Analyzer (DTSA), which runs on Macintosh family computers, and which is available for download from the US National Institute of Standards and Technology web site. DTSA incorporates routines for both SEM and TEM spectral evaluation.

At present, user interaction is required to optimize the various parameters of the model to achieve a good fit, so automatic batch processing of spectra is not possible. However, as we shall see in Chapter 6, the benefit extends not only to performing a high-precision background fit, but to deriving other very useful information, contributing in other ways to the analysis of the sample.

4.4 Deconvolution of overlapping peaks

So far we have discussed only cases in which the characteristic peaks do not overlap with each other. Nature being as it is, we cannot limit our analyses to these cases. There are many cases of peak overlaps, of which a few common examples include the K_β lines of the elements from Ti to Ge, which overlap with the K_α line of the next heavier element, the overlap between S K, Mo L and Pb M lines, or the extensive overlap between the L lines of adjacent and nearly adjacent rare-earth elements.

In some cases it may be possible to find enough information from elemental lines that do not suffer overlap. For example, in a Fe–Co alloy, the Fe K_β and the Co K_α lines overlap. It would be possible to quantify the results based on a comparison of the Fe K_α and the Co K_β lines. This would require the determination of the appropriate K factor, but the principal disadvantage is that the number of counts in the K_β line is only of the order of 12% of the intensity of the K_α line. Hence the precision of the analysis would be degraded, but may still be adequate for the purpose at hand.

More generally, it will be necessary to perform some sort of deconvolution of the overlapping lines. This obviously requires that the shapes and relative intensities of the sub-peaks be known. Fortunately, within a particular family of lines, the relative intensities of the various peaks are not a function of the electron energy – for example, the ratio of the K_α to K_β counts is constant for a particular element. (Note, though, that the same is not true for the ratios of one family to another.) However, the detector characteristics will change the line shapes. It is relatively simple to compensate for changes in the detector energy resolution as a function of system time constant, but more intractable is the problem of 'tailing' or incomplete charge collection. For this reason, it is best if the line shapes are derived from measured spectra obtained on the same instrument in the same analytical conditions and at about the same count rates as the unknown spectra. Even so, as we have seen in the preceding chapter, line shapes, and in particular incomplete charge collection, can vary over time even on a single system. However, good databases exist of the energies and relative intensities of lines for almost all elements in the periodic table, and, when using modern detectors in good condition, in which the incomplete charge collection has been reduced to very low levels, very satisfactory deconvolution results can usually be achieved by use of theoretically generated peak shapes. Most commercial analyser software packages make provision for such peak shape generation and for the recording and storage of experimental standards. In either case, though, it is critical that the amplifier gain and zero be correctly adjusted. Good deconvolution is precluded if the measured and standard spectra do not have the same centroids.

The most basic form of deconvolution is 'peak stripping'. Consider a steel containing Cr, Mn and Fe. The Cr K_β overlaps with the Mn K_α, and the Mn K_β overlaps with the Fe K_α. After background subtraction, the Cr K_α peak in the standard spectrum is normalized to the measured Cr K_α. The normalized Cr K peak is then subtracted, leaving the Mn and Fe. The process is repeated for the Mn peak, now leaving the stripped Fe for measurement. Although simple enough to be performed by hand, and illustrated as such in *Figure 4.5*, this process is not often implemented in commercial software, as more sophisticated regression procedures are easy to write and are less interactive. However, it is rather less sensitive to gain and zero errors than regression techniques.

Other cases of more complete peak overlap, as, for example, between Ti and Ba in $BaTiO_3$, illustrated in *Figure 4.6*, are intractable by peak stripping. In these cases, a regression analysis must be performed. This is

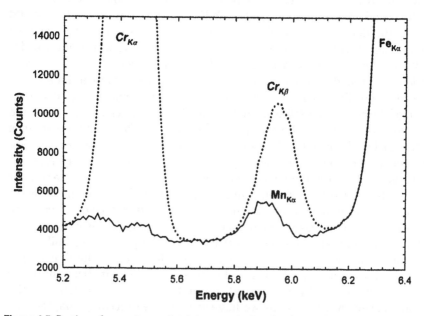

Figure 4.5. Portion of a spectrum of stainless steel, showing (dotted) the original Cr peak, and (solid) the spectrum after subtraction of a theoretical fit to the Cr peak. In the latter spectrum, the presence of a small peak due to Mn becomes visible. This processing was performed entirely by hand, and, while very satisfactory, was also very laborious.

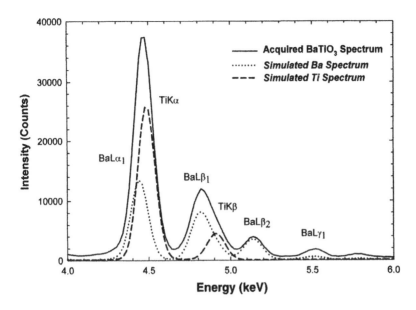

Figure 4.6. A measured spectrum from barium titanate, showing the region of the Ba L and Ti K peaks. Models of Ba and Ti spectra are overlaid. Analysis proceeds by performing a regression fit of the two models to the measured spectrum (after performing a background subtraction on the measured spectrum). The process also works if a top-hat filter has been applied to the measured and modelled spectra. It is important that the gain and zero, and the energy resolution of the measured spectrum match those of the model. It is usually advantageous to use measured standard spectra of the elements, rather than theoretical models as in our illustration, but this is not always possible.

implemented in some way in all modern software packages, and the exact details need not concern us here. We should reiterate, however, that accurate knowledge of peak shapes and gain and zero adjustments is critical for successful analysis – the more complete the overlap and the more subtle the difference between peaks (see e.g. the MoS_2 spectrum of *Figure 4.7*) the greater the possibility of the analysis producing incorrect results – sometimes wildly so. We should also add that quite modest improvements in spectral energy resolution can greatly improve the precision of a deconvolution. In later chapters we will show that in cases where peak overlap is not a problem, there is often advantage to be gained by trading processing time (and hence resolution) for count rate. If deconvolution is required, though, it will probably be better to trade at least some of the counts for better energy resolution. The analyst will have to examine each specific case to determine the best compromise, if the best precision in the result is vital.

Readers may wonder how the 'top-hat' filtering described above changes peak deconvolution. In fact, it has been shown that, provided the standard spectra and the unknown are subject to the same filter, deconvolution works exactly the same on the filtered spectra as on the raw spectra. Thus

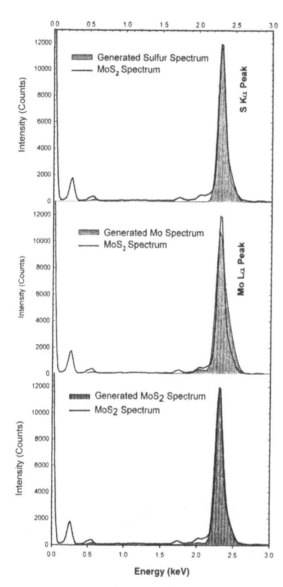

Figure 4.7. A spectrum from MoS_2, fitted with a modelled S peak (top), with Mo (centre) and with a modelled MoS_2 spectrum (bottom), showing how subtle the differences between the spectra are in this case. Nevertheless, without using extreme effort on the part of the operator, a commercial EDX quantification program was able to deconvolute the spectrum, giving a composition within about 5% of nominal for the compound.

filtering to remove the background, followed by an automatic peak search and a fitting of stored library spectra is an attractive, totally 'hands-off' analysis procedure which is reproducible and predictable – provided, as we shall again stress, that extreme care is taken with the preparation of the standard spectra and that the calibration of the detector is carefully maintained. As we have mentioned in Chapter 3, some manufacturers provide an electronic 'zero peak' which is saved with the spectrum and which records errors in the system zero setting, while also recording the actual energy resolution of the detector and analyser. In this way, two of the required preconditions of the analysis are satisfied.

The perspicacious reader may also wonder whether self-absorption of X-rays in the sample (an issue we will describe in detail in Chapters 5 and 6) can ever interfere with spectral deconvolution. The answer is that, indeed, it can. The example of a steel containing Cr, Mn and Fe is such a case. The Mn K_α line is lower in energy than the Cr K absorption edge, and so is not strongly absorbed in the Cr, while the K_β line of Mn is above the Cr absorption edge and is strongly absorbed. Hence the measured ratio of the Mn K_α to K_β X-rays in a thick foil of the alloy will not match that from a pure standard. This will lead to an error in the subtraction of the Mn K_β overlap from the Fe K_α peak. In this particular case, the error is not likely to be large, as the Cr content in a typical steel is likely to be only 20% or less, and the Mn content is typically of the order of a few per cent, so the absorption would be relatively small, leading to a small error in the correction to the Fe counts, which is itself small to begin with. The situation would be very different, though, if an analysis were being made on a Cr–20%Mn–5%Fe sample, for example. It should be mentioned that, unless accounted for as we shall describe in the following chapters, the self-absorption in the sample will generally lead to other, more serious errors in the analysis than these difficulties with deconvolution – certainly that would be true of the example we have used here.

In many cases of peak deconvolutions, the absorption edges do not interfere with the peaks being analysed. It should be obvious, though, that the overall quantitative analysis can still be affected by absorption, and the analyst must still consider thickness effects carefully.

4.5 Statistical considerations

So far, we have considered only determining the number of counts recorded in each X-ray peak. A quantitative analysis requires an estimate of the uncertainty of the measurement. There are a number of factors to consider.

4.5.1 *Poisson statistics*

The counting of X-rays obeys Poisson statistics. The interested reader is referred to any good book on statistics for a more complete discussion, but a brief summary will be helpful here.

Poisson statistics is, essentially, the statistics of positive integers. A system counting events (such as the arrival of X-rays) obeys Poisson statistics if a suitably small time interval can be defined such that the probability of detection of an event during that interval is much smaller than 1, and is independent of whether an event was detected during the preceding interval. Although we do not justify the statement here, X-rays do satisfy this criterion. The more familiar Gaussian statistics apply more generally, and in particular apply to continuous functions. However, for suitably large positive numbers (which actually means greater than about 25), Poisson statistics can be approximated by Gaussian statistics, and we shall follow the general practice of analysts in discussing statistical effects in terms of the latter.

4.5.2 Gaussian statistics

In Chapter 6, we derive an expected count rate I (in counts s^{-1}) for characteristic X-rays from an element in a thin sample. If we count for some extremely long time τ, we would find that the number of counts we measured would be approximately $I\tau$. Imagine, though, that we count for some shorter time, such that the product $I\tau$ is N, and that we repeat the experiment many, many times. We will in general record a different number of counts each experiment, though all the results should be reasonably close to N. What statistics tells us is that if we plot the number of times $P(N')$ a particular value N' is recorded, we will obtain a curve with a maximum (or centroid) at N, obeying the equation:

$$P = P_o e^{-\left(\frac{\delta}{\sigma}\right)^2}$$

(4.1)

where δ is $N_o - N'$, σ, the standard deviation, is equal to $\sqrt{N}$, and P_o is the number of times we record N counts. A characteristic of such a distribution is that 65% of the measurements will be within $\pm\ \sigma$ of N, 95% will be within $\pm\ 2\sigma$, and 99.5% will be within $\pm\ 3\sigma$.

Unfortunately, this is not the information we need. We make a single measurement N', and we need to estimate the probability that it is within a certain range of N. Fortunately, the statistics of reasonably large numbers again comes to our rescue, and it transpires that for N' larger than about 36, we can approximate that we have a 65% probability of being within $\pm\ \sqrt{N'}$ of N, 95% probability of being within $\pm\ 2\sqrt{N'}$, and so on.

4.6 The impact of statistics

Let us imagine we are performing an experiment, in which we have a sample consisting of approximately 90% element A, 10% element B, and we will assume that the number of counts acquired is in direct proportion to the concentration of the element in the sample. We require determination of this composition to within 1%, that is, our answer for B will be 9 ± 1%, with 99.5% certainty. How many counts must we acquire? An analytic determination is complex; we will make some simplifications here. There will be about nine times more counts from element A than element B. Imagine we have 900 counts from A, 100 from B. The measurement of N_A has a 99.5% probability of being within 90 counts of the expected value – about a 10% uncertainty. The measurement of N_B will have a 99.5% probability of being within 30 counts of the expected value – a 30% uncertainty.

Now the concentration of B in the sample is given by

$$C_B = \frac{100 \pm 30}{(900 \pm 90) + (100 \pm 30)} \qquad (4.2)$$

The minimum possible value of this expression is 70/1060, or 0.066, while the maximum value is 130/940, or 0.138. We see that the error is about 3.6%, which we notice is not greatly different from what we would have assumed had we merely taken the error of the measurement of element B, referenced to the actual measurement of B (i.e. 30% relative error of an absolute composition of 0.1 leads to an absolute error of 3%). In general, it is true that if a minor element is being measured against a major element, the statistical error in the measurement of the minor constituent dominates the overall error of the measurement.

Nevertheless, the error of 3.6% does not meet our requirements. We will need to acquire about 10 times more counts, or about 10 000 (by extending the counting time, increasing the beam current or measuring a thicker part of the sample, or a combination of the three) to approach the 1% precision goal. Unfortunately, all these possible ways of increasing the total counts have consequences for the analysis, as we will discuss in later sections.

Statistics also sets practical limits on the achievable precision of the analysis. To gain another order of magnitude in precision (i.e. measurement to within 0.1%), we would need to increase the signal by two orders of magnitude, to about 10^6 counts, in the case of our example. As a rough rule, the intensity of the major peak in a spectrum from a thin sample is about equal to the total background (in the SEM this ratio is generally less favourable), so altogether at least 2×10^6 counts must be acquired. Most modern detectors can count at 20 000 counts s^{-1}, so this acquisition would take 100 s if enough X-rays can be generated. This is a practical time. However, yet another order of magnitude gain in analytical precision would require 10 000 s acquisition; this is probably not a practical proposition, at least for routine analyses. Actually, as we shall discuss in later chapters, other problems prevent the achievement of better analytical precision, anyway. Additionally, if the sample is thin and the electron probe small, not enough X-rays will be generated to allow counting at this rate, and the precision of the analysis will degrade as a result.

4.7 The effect of the background

Before leaving the subject of statistics, it is necessary to discuss the effect of the bremsstrahlung background on the analysis. As we have seen, the electron-excited X-ray spectrum consists of the characteristic peaks superimposed on a continuum background, which must be subtracted before the number of counts in the peak can be determined. This creates two problems. The first is that the uncertainty in the number of counts in the peak is three times (or twice, depending on the certainty level the user is requiring) the square root of the peak plus background counts. Thus a peak of 25 counts on a background of 100 counts will have a standard deviation of 11 counts, resulting in a 99.5% confidence level of 33 counts. Even at 95% confidence, the 25 counts measured are only just significant.

It should be stressed that the problem described in the last paragraph is due to the statistical channel-by-channel variation in the number of X-rays recorded, and is not related to the subtraction of the background. It is important to understand, however, that, from a statistical point of view, subtraction has exactly the same effect as addition, in that it adds uncertainty to the result. If there is uncertainty in background subtraction, that increases the uncertainty in the peak intensity. Fortunately for the average analyst, extreme precision in background stripping only becomes important when quantitative analysis at levels close to the detection limit is being attempted. We can use a simple illustration to show this. Suppose that 1% of an element in an otherwise pure thin film matrix is being analysed. We will assume that the peaks are near to each other but not interfering, and, for the sake of this illustration, that the analytical sensitivities are the same. An example of such an analysis might be 1% Cr in Fe. Empirically we know that in pure Fe foils, the background is of the order of 1% of the Fe K_α line, over the typical width of the line in the observed spectrum. Thus the Cr K_α line will have about the same number of counts as the background. Hence, a 10% error in estimating the background under the Cr peak will result in a 10% error in the determination of the number of counts in the peak, but this will correspond to only a 0.1% absolute error in the analysis. As we have seen, this level of error is comparable with the best precision attainable by EDX analysis.

4.8 Analytical strategy

A very different issue, but nevertheless one vital to performance of quality analysis, is the correct identification of the various spectral lines and other features of the spectrum. It is easy for the analyst with preconceptions of the result to neglect to consider other possibilities, with potentially disastrous consequences. We would like to think that such mistakes are not made, but we know, from personal observation of respected analysts, that they are. It is of the greatest importance that the practitioner implements a strategy designed to minimize such errors, the most common of which, perhaps, is misidentification of a line by failure to consider the possibility that other, overlapping lines may be present.

Let us comment that every feature of a spectrum is, in principle, identifiable. Only when a fully self-consistent explanation has been derived for the entire spectrum should the identification be considered confirmed. Any inconsistency must have an explanation. For example, a peak will not be 'a couple of channels off' unless all the other peaks are also out of position. Likewise, a weakly excited peak will not be present unless the stronger peaks are also visible. Routines provided by the system manufacturer for location and identification of peaks should not be relied upon, except as a starting point for the investigation.

Elemental identification should begin with the major peak in the spectrum. All the lines for that element, including escape and sum peaks (when present) should then be located and noted. Identification should then proceed to the next most intense unattributed peak, and so on. Once all lines have been identified, as a check, it is wise to use a modelling program (such as DTSA) to simulate a spectrum. This may demonstrate inconsistencies in peak-height ratios, which reveal the presence of other, interfering, lines. Even if complete agreement is reached at this stage, the possibility of overlaps should not be overlooked. For example, the K lines of S and L lines of Mo overlap almost precisely. While in a high-resolution system with good counting statistics the peak shapes can be seen to be significantly different, with poorer resolution and less counts, it will be very difficult to tell them apart. In a TEM the K lines of Mo will be excited and visible, but in an SEM, if operated at 20 keV or below, this will not be the case. Sometimes it will be necessary to modify the conditions of the measurement, or even perform a completely new experiment, for the sole purpose of confirming such a peak identification. It is undoubtedly true that in some cases the significance, or likelihood, of a mistake in such an identification would be of so little consequence as to not justify the effort involved in confirming it. It is, of course, the prerogative of the analyst to make such a choice, but it is important that it is made after full consideration, and not out of ignorance.

After all other possibilities have been exhausted, it may still be found (in a spectrum with a large number of counts) that a few small features are unidentified. If the analysis was performed in the TEM, it may be that these are coherent bremsstrahlung. This may be confirmed by acquiring another spectrum from the same region of the sample, but with either the tilt or the beam voltage changed. In either case, the position, and perhaps the intensity, of the peaks will change if they are, indeed, the result of coherent bremsstrahlung.

In this section, we have discussed only identifying the peaks in the spectrum. We will discuss how quantitative information is derived in the chapters on SEM and TEM, to which we shall now proceed.

5 Energy-dispersive X-ray microanalysis in the scanning electron microscope

5.1 Introduction

EDX analysis in the SEM is, perhaps, the most common application of X-ray microanalysis. With care taken, it is possible to get very useful quantitative results from a wide range of materials. Unfortunately, it is also possible, especially for the novice, to misinterpret the data wildly. It is, therefore, critical that all users, not just those looking for accurate results, have a clear knowledge of the fundamentals of the technique, and the prerequisites for quality microanalysis. This contrasts, to some extent, with EDX microanalysis in the TEM, when, as we shall see in Chapter 6, some simplifications and approximations can be made, limiting – but not eliminating – the scope for major errors in interpretation. We will begin our discussion with a simple description of the SEM.

The SEM column forms a focused probe of electrons on the sample. The beam energy is adjustable in the range 1–30 keV or thereabouts, and the probe current is approximately in the range 10^{-8}–10^{-11} A. The probe diameter is typically in the range 1–10 nm (of course, all the values quoted here are generalizations). An image is formed by scanning the probe in a raster pattern on the sample, detecting some excited radiation from the sample, and storing the result either as a pattern of varying intensity levels on a cathode ray tube (CRT) screen (recorded, optionally, on film) or as a pattern of digital values in electronic memory for later manipulation and display. The scan may also be stopped, and the beam steered to a specific point on the sample surface, so that the emitted radiation from that point may be analysed in detail. In this chapter, we shall be implicitly describing operation of the instrument in this mode, analysing the resulting X-rays with the EDX detector.

As we discussed in Chapter 2, various different interactions may take place between an incident electron and atoms in the sample. In general, the results of any of these interactions are one or more electrons, with a total energy close to that of the incident electron, leaving the site of the interaction. These electrons, in turn, can interact with another atom, and so on, quickly leading to a complex cascade of events throughout a significant volume of the sample. While interactions between energetic electrons and lighter atoms are most likely to result in atomic electron excitations, after which the incident electron continues with only modestly reduced energy and in approximately the original direction, interactions with heavier atoms are increasingly more likely to result in elastic scattering of the incident electron through large angles, which can approach 180°. Electrons scattered through more than 90° are said to have been 'backscattered'.

The classic description of the interaction volume shows 'teardrop' shape, illustrated in *Figure 5.1*. It is possible to model the interactions in a computer program, and use Monte Carlo techniques to simulate the beam propagation, allowing the total interaction to be studied in more detail. Using such a method (we actually used Electron Flight Simulator, a commercial implementation of the Monte Carlo modelling program), it can be shown that only in lighter materials at higher beam voltages is this classical picture close to reality. For example, in *Figure 5.2a* we illustrate a simulation of 30 kV beam trajectories in magnesium carbonate. In contrast, in *Figure 5.2b* is shown a simulation of 8 kV electron propagation in Pb. It can be seen that in this case the overall shape is more spherical – because of the effect of the backscattered electrons. The different scales of the illustrations should also be noted – this is emphasized by *Figure 5.2c*, which is the same simulation as *Figure 5.2b*, but plotted on the same length scale as *Figure 5.2a*. It is obvious that the dimensions of the volume of the interaction can vary from a few tenths of a micron to many microns, depending on the beam energy and the material.

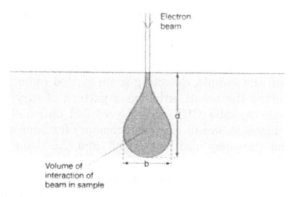

Figure 5.1. Sketch of the classic description of the interaction volume of the electrons in a SEM, and a 'teardrop' shape.

(a)

(b)

(c)

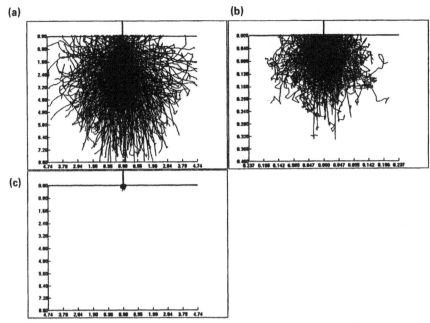

Figure 5.2. (a) Simulation of the electron path for 30 kV electrons in magnesium carbonate. (b) Simulation of the electron path for 8 kV electrons in Pb. (c) The same as (b), but plotted on the same scale as (a). Scales in µm.

While, as we have seen, individual electrons can follow widely different trajectories, the average behaviour of the beam is quite predictable and reproducible. The rate at which a beam loses energy with depth in the sample is well described by Bethe's equation:

$$\frac{dE}{dx} = -7.85 \cdot 10^4 \left(\frac{Z\rho}{AE_m}\right) \ln\left(\frac{1.66E}{J}\right) \text{keV cm}^{-1} \tag{5.1}$$

where E_m is the mean energy of the electrons, Z and A are respectively the mean atomic number and atomic weight of the sample, J is the mean ionization potential of the elements of the sample, and ρ is the sample density in g cm^{-2}.

SEM images are generally formed by detecting either the secondary (low-energy) electrons emitted from the sample, or the backscattered (high-energy) electrons. While secondary electrons can be formed anywhere within the volume of interaction, only those generated within a few nanometers of the surface actually escape to be detected. Most of these are generated before the beam spreads out, and thus provide information about a very small volume of material centred on the electron probe's point of impact on the surface. Backscattered electrons that re-emerge from the sample surface can also generate secondary electrons, but in most cases these are few enough, and sufficiently diffuse, that they do not mask the high-resolution detail in the main secondary electron signal.

The backscattered electrons able to escape from the sample are formed only in the first part of the electron trajectory, before the beam has lost too much energy, while they still stand a good probability of getting back to the surface, but still at greater depths than the secondary electrons. Hence the detected backscattered electrons originate from a larger volume of the sample than do the secondary electrons, and thus form an image of lower resolution.

Production of X-rays can take place at any depth where the electron beam has enough energy to ionize the atoms. The probability of X-ray production will vary with depth, in a way that will vary from element to element. The details of these processes will form the subject of discussion of a large portion of this chapter, but it is clear that the volume from which the X-rays originate is substantially the whole interaction volume of the electron beam. While the X-rays can be absorbed as they pass through the material of the sample, they have, in general, a much longer path than electrons, and so have a good probability of leaving the sample and reaching the detector. Thus the spatial resolution of the X-ray signal is variable, and is frequently of the order of a micron or more. We give a graphic illustration of this effect in Chapter 7, where we show the difference between X-ray maps acquired from the same area of a sample, at different beam voltages.

We will conclude this introduction by making a few remarks about the electron microprobe. In principle, the electron microprobe is simply an SEM, on which has been mounted one (or, more usually, several) crystal X-ray spectrometers. The crystal spectrometers detect the X-rays with far higher energy resolution than does the EDX detector. While the resulting improved peak-to-background certainly contributes to the improved sensitivity of the microprobe, it is not the main factor. As we saw in Chapter 3, the maximum count rate of the EDX detector is limited to a few thousand counts per second. The crystal spectrometers, in contrast, can count much faster, thus providing better statistics in the X-ray analysis. However, this count rate can only be achieved if enough X-rays are generated in the sample. The electron beam currents typical of SEM imaging are not adequate to generate these count rates. Therefore the electron column of the microprobe is designed to produce electron probes with far more current, and correspondingly larger probe sizes, than the SEM. It is also necessary that the probe current be extremely stable over the time of the measurement (because the data acquisition in the microprobe is serial in nature, and the conditions must remain the same over the time of the experiment). This requirement, too, introduces some design constraints into the system.

It is possible to obtain a secondary or backscattered electron image of most samples in either an SEM or an electron microprobe; the image formed by the SEM may be of higher resolution, but in many cases the resolution of the microprobe image will be adequate. Likewise, a sample can be analysed in either instrument. The result from the microprobe will have higher sensitivity and precision, but often the data obtained in the SEM will be adequate.

Typical uses of the electron microprobe and the SEM are different. The purpose of the microprobe is to obtain high-quality quantitative analytical information; the user accepts that, in order to reach this goal, specific, high-quality specimen preparation is required. Generally, rough samples are not acceptable. On the other hand, the SEM user wants to relate composition to features of the sample surface – facets, for example. Grinding and polishing are out of the question. The microanalysis must be performed on the sample 'as is'. As we shall see, this limits the achievable quality of the microanalytical data. While the microprobe user will be very concerned about the details of the spectral processing in order to maximize the precision of the analysis, this is simply not worthwhile for many SEM samples, as the prerequisites for precise analysis (which we shall describe in the following sections) are not satisfied.

5.2 Fundamentals of X-ray analysis in the SEM

Let us for now assume that the region of the sample we wish to analyse is homogeneous over the region surrounding the point of impact of the electron beam. Let us consider what happens before X-rays reach the detector and are collected to form a spectrum. For the purpose of our discussion, we will assume that the sample has two components of significantly different atomic number. An Ni–Al alloy would be an example of such a material. The Ni K_α line is at about 7.48 keV, and the L lines are at about 0.85 keV, while the Al K line is at about 1.49 keV.

A typical electron energy selected for such an analysis might be 20 keV. When the electron beam penetrates the surface of the sample, the voltage is about optimum for exciting the Ni K X-rays, but is well above the optimum for exciting the Al K or Ni L X-rays. As the electrons propagate through the sample and lose energy, the production of Ni K X-rays decreases with depth. However, the production of the Al K and Ni L X-rays increases, because the beam energy is getting closer to the optimum energy for production of these X-rays. Eventually the production of Ni K X-rays will cease, once the beam energy reaches about 8 keV (the K ionization energy for Ni), but the production of Al K and Ni L X-rays will still be increasing. Only at some greater depth still will the production of these X-rays peak, and then quite rapidly drop to zero. The process is illustrated by the simulations (once again, generated by Electron Flight Simulator) shown in *Figure 5.3*, where we present a model of this experiment. Of course, the details will vary if the initial beam voltage is changed. For example, if the beam voltage is 10 keV, then almost no Ni K X-rays will be generated, and the production of the Al K and Ni L X-rays will be less than half as deep as in the first example (because higher-energy electrons lose energy more slowly than lower-energy ones, so the total range of 10 keV electrons is less than half the range of 20 keV ones).

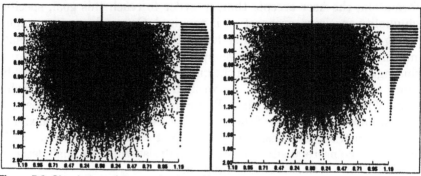

Figure 5.3. Simulation of the production of K-shell X-rays of Al (left) and Ni (right) from a sample of NiAl in the SEM at 20 kV.

In this description, we have assumed that the electron beam loses energy smoothly (according to the Bethe equation, for example). There is a short-coming to this approach, however, because although the Bethe equation may accurately predict the *average* energy of the electrons, it does not say anything about the energy spread. In fact this can be quite large, with some significant fraction of the electrons penetrating relatively large distances without losing much energy, and others actually being scattered back towards the surface, adding to the electron intensity, but increasing the energy spread of the electrons there. Some of these electrons can excite Ni K X-rays (in our example above) more deeply in the sample than our simple description would suggest, and in general, the whole plot of X-ray production will be less well defined. However, the general principle of the description is completely valid, and shows that the production of X-rays in a sample in the SEM is not a simple function of the composition of the sample.

Having been generated, the X-rays must reach the X-ray detector before they can contribute to the spectrum. We discussed in Chapter 3 the sensitivity of the detector itself, and the fact that only a finite (small) number of the total X-rays produced actually enter it, because of geometrical considerations. We must also consider how the X-rays interact with the sample. *Figure 5.4* illustrates the problem. As we saw in Chapter 2, X-rays can be absorbed as they pass through matter; the absorption being a very strong function of the identity of the absorber and the energy of the X-ray, and is not monotonic with energy. In *Figure 5.5*, for example, we show the mass absorption coefficients for Ni and Al as a function of X-ray energy, on a linear scale, with the energies of the Ni K and L lines and the Al K line indicated. This illustration was derived from the parameterized equations published by Heinrich; we shall have more to say about such sources later in this chapter.

To return to our example of analysis of NiAl, let us imagine that the X-ray detector axis is at an angle of 40° to the horizontal plane (a typical

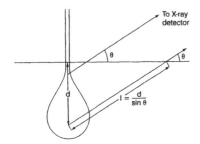

Figure 5.4. Sketch showing the various interactions that can take place between generated X-rays and the sample material.

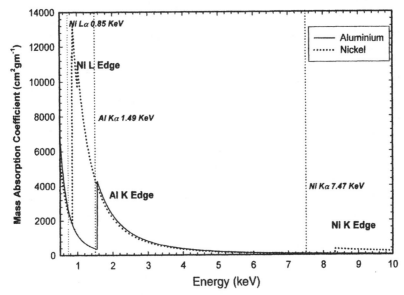

Figure 5.5. Model of the X-ray mass absorption coefficients of Ni and Al as a function of X-ray energy. The energies of the Ni K_α and L_α and the Al K_α lines are also indicated.

value, and exactly that of the X-ray detector in the SEM used to generate our examples here). Consider an Al K_α X-ray generated 1 μm below the surface, and travelling initially towards the detector. In its path it must pass through 1.6 μm of the material of the sample. Using the information given in Chapter 2, and mass absorption coefficients computed from Heinrich's parameterization, we can calculate that the X-ray will have only about 8% probability of reaching the surface, and thus actually arriving at the detector. In contrast a Ni K_α X-ray generated at the same depth would have 94% probability of reaching the detector. (The alert reader will object that the probability of such an X-ray being generated will be very small; this indeed is true. Our purpose here, though, is to illustrate the very large differences in absorption that can exist between different X-rays.) Even the

Ni L X-ray at 850 eV, generated at the same depth, will have a 17% probability of being detected. Of course, the fraction of the various X-rays that reaches the detector will vary by the depth at which they are generated.

It is probably obvious to the reader, but, for completeness, we will point out that the effect of absorption is strongly dependent on the tilt of the sample surface with respect to the X-ray detector. This is, of course, because the path length of the X-rays in the sample depends upon this tilt, as can be seen in the diagram of *Figure 5.6*.

Figure 5.7 illustrates extreme examples of the foregoing effects. The specimen was a Ni–49.3at%Al coupon, kindly made available by B. Pint. The figure overlays a spectrum obtained at 30-kV beam energy from a flat area of the surface (the solid line), with a similar spectrum obtained from a protrusion on the surface (dotted line), and a spectrum obtained from the flat area at 10-kV beam energy (the dashed line). Qualitatively, the differences are obvious. The reader can probably deduce that the dotted spectrum was obtained from the side of the protrusion facing away from the X-ray detector; the X-rays had, therefore, to travel through the thickness of the protrusion to reach the detector. We will discuss these spectra again later in this chapter.

There is yet another problem the analyst must contend with. As we saw in Chapter 2, the main result of the absorption of an X-ray in an atom of matter is the generation of a core-level vacancy in the electronic structure. This event can be the precursor to the generation of a new characteristic X-ray from the atom, which will, of course, be one of the atomic species of interest in the sample. The process is called X-ray fluorescence. By it, the intensity of some of the lines in the spectrum can be enhanced. Clearly, the fluoresced X-ray can only be of lower energy than the fluorescing X-ray. As a general rule, the fluorescence will be stronger the less the difference between the energy of the fluorescing X-ray and the ionization energy of the vacancy that leads to the fluoresced X-ray, and obviously the magnitude of the effect will depend on the intensity of the fluorescing X-ray (and hence on the concentration of the fluorescing element in the sample). This effect can be quite serious because, although only a very small fraction of the

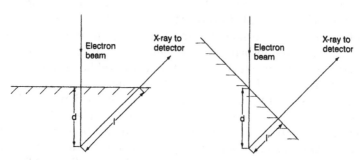

Figure 5.6. The path length of X-rays in the sample as a function of the sample tilt.

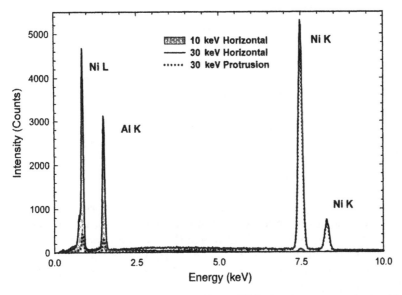

Figure 5.7. Overlaid spectra of NiAl acquired in an SEM, showing spectra obtained from a flat surface and a protrusion at 30 kV, and from the same flat surface at 10 kV. The spectra from the flat surface match each other well at low voltage because the excitation probability of the X-rays is very low. Conversely, the two spectra acquired at 30kV beam voltage match at higher energies, but the low energy X-rays are absorbed strongly by the sample protrusion, leading to severe attenuation of the spectrum in this region.

original characteristic X-rays travel towards the X-ray detector, all the X-rays can potentially lead to fluorescence. Of course, only those fluoresced X-rays that are emitted towards the detector can potentially be detected, provided that they, in turn, are not absorbed by the sample.

In our example, we have seen that most of the Ni K X-rays that are travelling in a direction towards the sample surface will not be absorbed. However, most of the Ni K X-rays moving into the sample will eventually lead to the generation of an Al K or Ni L ionization, and perhaps an X-ray. The chances are, though, that this will be so far into the sample that these X-rays will be reabsorbed (a corollary of the low absorption of the Ni K X-ray is that its path length in the sample is large), and will not, therefore, contribute to the Ni L or Al peaks. The case of the Al X-rays, though, is quite different. They are absorbed relatively strongly by the Ni, and so travel only a short distance. Since they are generated relatively deeply in the sample, X-rays travelling in all directions, and not only those travelling into the sample, contribute to the fluorescence. Finally, the chances of the resulting Ni L X-ray being able to reach the detector are fairly good. Hence the Ni L X-ray peak can be strongly enhanced by fluorescence from the Al X-rays. For quantitative microanalysis, it is imperative that this fluorescence be taken into account in processing the spectrum.

5.3 Quantitative microanalysis in the SEM

The reader who has stayed with our discussion up to this point may, perhaps, be forgiven for wondering whether there is any point in continuing. After all, if there are so many difficulties, each dependent on so many variables, how do we move forward?

It is, in fact, true that a good many users of EDX analysis in the SEM do not need high-quality quantitative analysis. To illustrate the point, earlier in the very day on which we were writing this section of text, we were helping a user whose sample consisted of a mixture of MnO_2 and Sb powders; he needed to know the relative sizes of the particles of each constituent. Clearly no 'quantitative' analysis was required – each particle's composition could be only one or the other of the ingredients. Nevertheless, many other applications of the technique do require a more or less precise statement of the composition. For these cases, some processing of the raw data must obviously be undertaken before the final result can be determined.

It is a tribute to two generations of researchers that in fact the electron microprobe has become one of the most trusted tools available to the microanalyst. All the various problems we have discussed have been researched, documented and analysed, and workable models have been developed to permit correction of analytical data to within about 0.1% absolute or better (depending on the circumstances of the particular analysis). These models are applicable directly to EDX analysis in the SEM (although, as we have seen, the limited count rate of the EDX detector constrains the ultimate sensitivity and precision of the analysis). In some ways, the EDX analyst has an advantage over the microprobe worker, as the X-ray detector is far more predictable and stable (the crystal spectrometers of the microprobe require daily re-characterization, and each spectrometer has a unique response, unlike other, even nominally identical instruments), and, since the spectra are obtained in parallel, rather than with sequential scanning as in the microprobe, the demands on the stability of the electron source are greatly reduced. All models, however, have some immutable requirements: the sample must either be homogeneous (over regions large compared with the analysis volume), polished, flat and mounted in the instrument in a precisely known orientation (usually perpendicular to the beam), or of some other, equally precisely defined geometry.

5.3.1 ZAF correction

The *ZAF* correction is by far the most widely used correction scheme for microprobe and SEM–EDX analysis, and is the only one that will be given more than passing mention here. The basic scheme, which is applicable to polished, flat, homogeneous samples, was first proposed by Castaing (1951), although it has been substantially refined since. Our description here is, of course, a simplified understanding of the method. In particular, the theory of the various corrections will not be addressed.

We start by assuming that no correction is necessary, and the concentration of element i is simply given by the ratio of I_i, the measured characteristic X-ray intensity from element i, to $I_{(i)}$, the intensity from a pure sample of the element analysed under identical conditions:

$$C_i = \frac{I_i}{I_{(i)}} \qquad (5.2)$$

Starting from the composition so derived, a correction is first applied to compensate for the difference in X-ray generation (including the distribution with depth, and also allowing for backscattered electrons) because the mean atomic number Z of the sample is different from the pure element; next, from the depth distribution is computed an absorption correction A, and finally a fluorescence correction F is applied, so that

$$C_i = [Z.A.F]\,\frac{I_i}{I_{(i)}} \qquad (5.3)$$

From the corrected composition, a second set of corrections is derived to refine the composition further, and so on until a desired degree of convergence in the result is achieved. Corrections for differences in crystal efficiency, detector sensitivity, and so on, are inherently included in the procedure. Provision is also made in refinements to the model for the use of compound standards, in addition to the pure-element standards we have described. The calculations are readily programmed into a computer, and are generally available at the click of a mouse button in modern commercial software.

A feature of the method is that it generates the concentration of each element within the analysed volume without a normalization step – in other words, no assumption is made that the total 'composition' of the sample is 100%. If the method has been appropriately applied, then the sum of all the components should, of course, be 100%. Hence a built-in check on the calculations is available – if the computed sum of the components is incorrect, then an error has been made, and the results are not trustworthy. We should note that the converse is not true – a computed sum of 100% does not guarantee an accurate analysis. It is possible that errors have been made which happen to cancel in the calculated sum.

We note also that it is critical that all the atoms in the sample must be accounted for in the calculations, even if they do not produce a useful X-ray signal. This is because both the electron propagation and X-ray absorption are functions of all the atomic species present, not just those contributing to the X-ray signal. For the analysis of oxides, for example, it is usual to assume the O content from stoichiometry.

Although we are not describing the detailed theory of the corrections, it is important that we mention their limitations. The *ZAF* correction requires a knowledge of the absorption of all the X-rays of interest and the electron range in the sample, together with corrections for backscattered electrons and fluorescence. We have commented on how well the theory provides a spectral correction, but it is still imperfect. Even for values that are amenable to measurement (such as mass absorption coefficients), it is impossible to measure the absorption of all possible X-rays in all absorbers. To address the problem, parameterized equations, based on theoretical models of the physics, have been derived. The parameters are determined by fitting measured values, where available. Unknown values can then be predicted by solving the equations with the appropriate variables (atomic number or atomic weight, for example). The parameterized mass absorption coefficient equations of Heinrich, referred to earlier in this chapter, and in Chapter 2, are such a set of equations. It will be clear to the reader that the values derived from these equations are necessarily approximations, and in some cases (because of errors in earlier measurements, typographical errors in tables of values propagated from before the days of computerized data recording, etc.) may be significantly in error. Although the *ZAF* correction is remarkably good (considering how many factors are involved and their complexity), it is still vital that the researcher confirm that it is sufficiently reliable for the particular combination of elements under investigation and the purpose for which the analysis is being performed. Although we are anticipating the next section, we will add that standardless *ZAF* analysis depends upon still more properties that are derived from parameterized equations (the ionization cross section and the fluorescence yield, which we described in Chapter 2), and is thus more prone to uncertainties.

5.3.2 Standardless ZAF correction

The *ZAF* method of correction, in its original form, was a correction based on a series of initial experimentally determined quantities (the intensities of the X-ray signals from the various standard samples). The long-term stability of the crystal spectrometers and the detectors cannot be assured (because of details we have not discussed), nor can their sensitivity be readily predicted. Therefore these initial standard measurements must take place as part of the same experimental session as the investigation of the unknown sample, and certainly cannot be replaced by any theoretically deduced standardization. However, when using the EDX detector, it is possible, because of its relative predictability and stability, and the parallel mode of spectral acquisition, to make some simplifications.

Firstly, it is possible to assume that the detector sensitivity does not vary with time. This allows a single measurement of a standard spectrum to be stored and used at a future time. Provided the beam currents used to obtain both the standard and unknown spectra are recorded, then the spectra can be normalized, and the *ZAF* method may be applied. We take for granted that other aspects of the analysis (beam voltage and sample position, for example) are identical in all cases.

Since the beam current is simply a scaling factor for the analysis, then by normalizing the final concentration to 100%, the need to measure the current during the analysis can be eliminated, at the expense, of course, of the built-in consistency check which we discussed in the preceding section. Since measurement of the beam current with the precision required to be useful is difficult, this is a significant experimental simplification.

When stored standards are used, as we have described in the last two paragraphs, the analysis is still restricted to elements, and beam conditions, for which the stored standards have been generated. In fact, the various physical effects that determine the X-ray spectrum are so thoroughly researched and understood that a very good approximation of the X-ray signal expected from many solids can be obtained purely from theory. The huge advantage of this method is that a standard spectrum can be generated 'on the fly' for any desired microscope conditions, regardless of whether a similar sample has ever been analysed before. The disadvantage is the added degree of uncertainty in the result, which we described at the end of the preceding section. Since no standard samples are used, this mode of spectral analysis is called, logically enough, 'standardless *ZAF* analysis'.

If a sample of known composition, close to that of the unknown, is available, then it can be used to 'tweak' the standardless parameters to give an improved correction, though it is important, of course, that the known sample be reliable and free of artifacts. It is easy in many cases to reach the limit of precision set by the counting statistics, and it is futile, obviously, to attempt any closer correction. Conversely, in the absence of such a standard, and especially if a completely new chemical system is being investigated, it is impossible to be sure that the theoretical computations are acceptably accurate.

The SEM quantification software packages offered by manufacturers of all modern EDX systems include an implementation of standardless *ZAF* correction. It is the mode of analysis employed almost universally by novice and 'casual' SEM users, and in fact is capable, as we shall see from the example spectra we give later in this chapter, which were corrected by our relatively modern commercial system, of very satisfactory performance.

5.3.3 *Other correction methods*

The name '*ZAF* correction' is a little confusing, because it is, at the same time, a description of what corrections must be made to the data, and a particular algorithm for performing the correction. Other algorithms are possible, one such being the $\phi(\rho, z)$ method, which starts from a model of the production of X-rays as a function of depth in the sample, and then performs the absorption and fluorescence corrections, as well as allowing for the contribution of backscattered electrons. All such corrections must allow for the same effects that we have already described, and indeed use the same basic physical descriptions. Only the details of the calculations are different. We will, therefore, not discuss these methods further, other than to say that, at least at the present stage of implementation, none of them appears to offer any overwhelming advantage in reliability over the classic *ZAF* correction.

In special cases, for example where standards of known composition, similar to the unknown, are available (a situation common for the geologist, to whom a vast library of thoroughly well-characterized standards is usually available), then great simplifications of the foregoing are possible. In these cases, it is relatively easy to determine a composition difference between two samples limited only by the counting statistics. The protocol for these types of experiments is usually developed locally, and will be very dependent upon the details of the analysis being performed.

5.4 Semi-quantitative microanalysis in the SEM

5.4.1 Discussion

By 'quantitative analysis' we mean a composition stated with analytically derived precision. Uncertainties in the typical SEM sample, specifically its surface topography and compositional homogeneity, make it impossible to specify the precision of any analytical result we may derive from a measured X-ray spectrum. By our definition, then, we cannot perform quantitative analysis in such cases. In our laboratory at least, most X-ray microanalysis performed in the SEM is, at best, 'semi-quantitative' in nature. In general, we would classify as 'semi-quantitative' any analysis which depended in any way on some non-quantifiable input, regardless of the 'experience' of the operator, who may (with complete justification) believe that, the uncertainty notwithstanding, the analysis is still 'reasonably accurate'. Some would argue that there is no such thing as a 'semi-quantitative' analysis – the result either is or is not quantitative. We would counter that by pointing out that there is a place in research for the 'educated guess' or the 'gut feeling'. Likewise, we would suggest that there is a place for the 'best effort' attempt at quantifying an analysis. The important – indeed, critical – thing is to recognize that scientific judgment has been employed in reaching the result.

Indeed, as we have already observed, in many cases the analyst does not need a 'quantitative' result, but can nevertheless derive a lot of useful information about the sample. A simple determination that, for example, element A is concentrated in a particular set of structures might suffice. By intelligent use of the image, and any other information at hand, and with an understanding of how the relationship between the beam, the sample and the detector affects the X-ray analysis, we can usually make an estimate of how closely the sample approximates the ideal, and how errors might affect our particular measurement. We can, if we choose, refine our knowledge of our particular system by analysing samples of known composition, analysing different areas of the sample that can be seen to have different characteristics or using other strategies appropriate to the analytical situation. By making educated use of information derived in this way, we can often draw very useful (and perfectly valid) conclusions.

A user will often run a quantitative routine (usually, standardless *ZAF*) on a spectrum from some feature in a sample that clearly does not meet the requirements for quantitative analysis. When asked to defend this, they will answer that the 'corrected' result is a closer approximation to the real analysis than can be obtained by just looking at the spectrum. On one hand, there is some logic to this argument; the 'correction' will allow, for example, for major differences in the excitation of different X-ray lines because of the beam energy. Certainly, if a sample is known to be generally flat and 'about' horizontal, then the quantitative analysis routines can be expected to yield a rough approximation of the composition. On the other hand, there is no legitimate scientific basis, in the general case, to taking this step. Indeed, it is easy to demonstrate cases where the 'corrected' analysis is further from the real composition than the simple ratio of peak heights. As a general rule, we strongly discourage our users from using the 'quantitative analysis' function of our software without having significant justification from the details of the experiment.

When running quantitative analysis routines, it is vital that the software be using the correct value for the incident beam energy. The analyst must set this up in the software at the appropriate time. In some cases, it must be done before a spectrum is acquired. One system, at least, known to the authors, stubbornly refuses to accept a new value for the incident beam energy for a spectrum, if it has been inadvertently saved with an incorrect value. Only by going through extensive manipulations can the software be made to accept the correction. Most systems include the beam voltage in the printout (or display) of the results. The analyst should make a habit of confirming that the software did, in fact, use the correct voltage.

The EDX spectrum can actually be used to measure the beam energy. The Kramers equation for the bremsstrahlung generation (Equation 2.1) tells us that the bremsstrahlung tends to zero at the beam energy. Furthermore, the approach to zero is not asymptotic, but the function crosses the axis at a well-defined gradient (in fact, the plot is asymptotic to -1 at very large Es). Thus if the spectrometer is set to display the X-ray energy range 0–40 keV, and a spectrum is obtained for a very extended period (because the bremsstrahlung intensity is very low in this region), then the energy at which the bremsstrahlung reaches zero (which is called the 'Duane–Hunt limit') is readily ascertained. This determination is quite precise because the X-ray spectrum is readily (and, hopefully, routinely) calibrated to within a few electron volts. *Figure 5.8* shows such a determination. The SEM was a modern, field-emission SEM in high-vacuum mode, the sample was a piece of tantalum. The high-voltage control was set to 8.0 kV, but it is clear from the figure that the actual accelerating voltage was 8.07 kV. As we shall see, an error of even this small magnitude can introduce a significant error in an X-ray analysis, depending on the

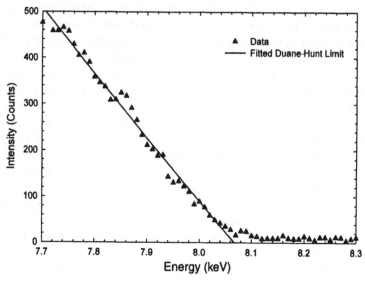

Figure 5.8. Illustration of a spectrum from solid Ta, showing the Duane–Hunt limit. The microscope was set for 8.0 keV, but the real energy can be seen to be about 8.07 keV.

conditions. We note, in passing, that the small 'tail' of counts recorded at energies above the Duane–Hunt limit is caused by such processes as the coincidence of two bremsstrahlung X-rays creating a sum event.

It is vital even when performing semi-quantitative analysis to allow for all the elements present in the sample when applying the correction routines, for the reasons we mentioned in Section 5.3.1. It is particularly easy to overlook this requirement when analysing oxides.

Despite what we said earlier in this section, if one is careful about the use of the 'quantify' button, the results can be extremely useful, as we shall see in a later sub-section. With thought, and perhaps a little experimentation, the analyst can get a 'feel' for how well the routines are working, and how prone the particular system under investigation is to error. While this may not satisfy an organization performing work to international standards committee certification requirements, it can certainly lead, in a less demanding environment, to a greatly expanded insight into the properties of the sample.

A final caveat to the subject of semi-quantitative analysis: if the quantification subroutine has been invoked, the end result is always a computer printout, with several significant figures, almost certainly with an error estimation, and all sorts of other numbers which have been used in the calculations. It is amazing how hard it is, intellectually, to ignore all those numbers, and to understand that the prerequisites for precise analysis, which were assumed by the computer's algorithm, simply were not met. This is not an issue with the computer's software, but with human nature, especially if the first result printed out is conveniently close to the anticipated one.

5.4.2 *Fingerprinting*

A completely different example of semi-quantitative analysis involves a technique called 'fingerprinting'. As applied to X-ray analysis, we mean not that we are attempting to derive a precise analysis of the sample, but that we can answer the question 'given an array of results from known samples, which one most closely resembles the result from the unknown?' An extremely simple (but nevertheless valid) example of a fingerprinting experiment would be the identification of MnO_2 and Sb particles that we mentioned in Section 5.3. The appropriate protocol is probably obvious to the reader. In general, a fingerprinting protocol involves the development of a specific set of sample and data acquisition requirements, so that every sample is prepared in the same way. A library of example data is then constructed from the desired set of known samples. Criteria for data matching are then derived (typically, from further research), so that one can state how well the unknown matches the selected standard. The protocol will obviously be highly specific to the application. Fingerprinting makes no attempt to perform a quantitative chemical analysis, but relies on the fact that two samples of the same composition, when prepared and analysed in exactly the same way, will yield exactly the same spectrum. Differences between the spectra can then be assumed to be significant, and appropriate deductions can be drawn from the observations.

5.4.3 *Examples*

It has been implicit in the discussion of the preceding section that, when performing semi-quantitative analysis, the operator makes sure that the sample is 'reasonably' flat and appropriately oriented in the microscope. To illustrate what we mean, let us return to the example of *Figure 5.7*. The sample of Ni–49.3at%Al was sliced from a rod, using a conventional diamond saw. The sides of the slice were quite shiny, and seemed to be parallel, but no measurement was made to confirm this. After cleaning, the sample was simply mounted on a specimen stub and put in the microscope. With the microscope stage set to zero tilt, an X-ray spectrum was acquired from a flat area free of obvious large scratches (the solid line in *Figure 5.7*) and analysed by the built-in automatic routines of the (modern) commercial system. The result was Ni–50.8at%Al. Spectra (not illustrated) were obtained with the sample tilted about 4° away from, and 6° towards, the X-ray detector. Without altering the conditions set up in the software, the results of the analysis of these spectra were respectively 47.7at%Al and 54.1at%Al. The dashed spectrum from *Figure 5.7*, obtained at a nominal beam energy of 10 kV was then subject to the same automatic analysis (allowing, of course, for the change in beam voltage). The result was 47.4at%Al. The data were obtained on the same microscope in which we showed the high voltage to be about 1% high, as described above. If we assume the same relative error at 10 kV, and analyse the spectrum specifying that the beam energy was 10.1 kV, the Al concentration is now given as 49.7at%, illustrating the importance of an accurate knowledge of the beam energy. (The excellent agreement between this result and the actual, known composition is totally fortuitous – the statistical error in this case is about ± 1%.)

We can deduce from these measurements that it is possible to get quite good analytical results rather easily, at least in some cases. However, we can also see that an error of 1° in the X-ray take-off angle would cause a change of 0.6% in the apparent Al composition. Such a change could be caused (with geometry of this system) by a height error in the sample of 0.4 mm, or by the X-ray detector being out-of-position by this amount (which could be caused, in turn, by a 0.1° error during machining some flange of the microscope chamber or X-ray detector assembly). It could also be caused by any number of other small errors. If we were meticulous in reproducing every detail of our analytical configuration in analysing another sample of Ni–Al, we could probably get a very good comparison between this standard sample and our unknown. However, had this sample been the unknown, we would not have been justified in saying anything more precise than that the composition was 'about Ni–50at%Al'. This is a good point at which to mention as an aside, that most microscopes give a readout of the sample 'height' (in reality, the distance from some relatively arbitrary position in the lens), derived from the excitation of the lenses. This reading is a useful aid to consistent operation, but should be checked for reproducibility at a variety of operating voltages and probe sizes. On our SEM, for example, this reading varies by about 0.1 mm over a wide range of operating conditions.

Returning to the Ni–Al, in contrast to the foregoing, the spectrum shown dotted in *Figure 5.7* was analysed as though it was obtained from a flat area of the sample. The result was 12.2at%Al. On the other hand, another spectrum (again not illustrated), taken from the side of the protrusion facing the X-ray detector, gave an analysis, via the automatic routines, of 60.9at%Al. These are, of course, extreme cases, but they do show the magnitude of the error that can be introduced by failure to take thoughtful consideration of the condition of the sample being analysed.

As an example of fingerprinting, consider the analysis of gunshot residue, which could, in all likelihood, be of interest to a forensic expert. In this case, the protocol might include the analysis of the range of particle sizes, but we will consider only the chemical analysis. The elements of interest would usually be Pb, Ba and Sb. A set of criteria for the relative numbers of counts in the peaks of these elements would be developed. Obtaining spectra from the unknown residues and comparison with the criteria would then provide a very simple determination of whether the unknown particles were gunshot residue or not. This is illustrated in *Figure 5.9*. A more complete database of characteristics could potentially allow a determination of the type of ammunition, manufacturer, and so on.

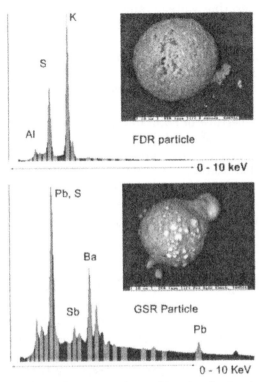

Figure 5.9. Illustration of analysis of gunshot residue showing two types of residue from control experiments. A series of windows are defined in the spectra (as shown), and the number of counts obtained in each of these windows from an unknown sample would be compared with these and other controls to determine which (if any) had a matching composition (illustration courtesy of D. L. Johnson, Z. Henneman and T. McGinn SUNY, ESF).

5.4.4 Conditions for X-ray microanalysis in the SEM

We will conclude this section with a short summary, in the form of a checklist, of the things the microanalyst must consider while working at the microscope.

- While inserting the specimen: determine the sample orientation, optimize as possible (either level, or in a predetermined orientation with respect to the detector); note area of interest.
- After inserting sample and obtaining electron image: switch off IR chamberscope (if fitted) – the IR radiation will interfere with most thin-window or windowless EDX detectors (in some microscopes this step is performed automatically).
- Check height of sample is at the correct position.
- If the X-ray detector is retractable, check that it is inserted to the proper position.

- Select the operating voltage, and check that the same voltage is correctly entered into the EDX software, so that it will be recorded with the spectra.
- Select appropriate processor time constant – short for high-count-rate applications such as X-ray mapping, or when peak overlaps are not a problem, long for best results when deconvolution is required.
- Adjust beam current (by changing probe size setting on microscope or intermediate aperture, or both) to obtain optimum count rate (ideally, dead time should be about 30–40%, but this cannot always be achieved because of other constraints of the experiment).
- Select a suitable area of the sample.
- Select an appropriate acquisition time, so that enough counts are obtained to give the required precision in the analysis, without spending time collecting unnecessary data.

5.5 EDX analysis in the VP-SEM and ESEM

So far we have discussed X-ray microanalysis in the high-vacuum, or conventional, SEM. A relatively recent development allows samples to be examined in a modest pressure of gas (usually water vapour). The pressure is typically below 1 torr in the variable-pressure (VP)-SEM, and up to 10 torr or even higher in the environmental SEM (ESEM). The latter instrument is currently protected by patents, and is made only by a single company. The former is offered, in various forms, by several manufacturers. The advantage of this type of microscope is that, within limits, it is possible to image insulating samples without the application of a conductive coat (because ions produced by the interaction of the beam with the gas in the chamber can neutralize any charge build-up on the sample), and it is also possible, within some limits, to perform *in situ* experiments, observing the processes as they take place. For reasons we need not enumerate here, microanalysis is not often useful for the *in situ* experiments. However, there is frequently the need to perform microanalysis on insulating samples. All the discussion of analysis in the high-vacuum microscope applies equally to the VP-SEM and the ESEM. Here we will discuss the additional problems that arise in this type of instrument.

There are two main difficulties. Of these two major problems, the better known is the scattering of the electron beam by the gas in the chamber. The working of the microscope, indeed, depends on this happening. Not all electrons are scattered – the ones that reach the sample without interacting with the gas form the high-resolution image. The electrons that are scattered are typically deflected far enough that they hit the sample away from the electron probe, and simply contribute a featureless background to the image intensity. This is illustrated in *Figure 5.10*. The resulting 'background' to the image intensity is subtracted electronically, leaving a high-

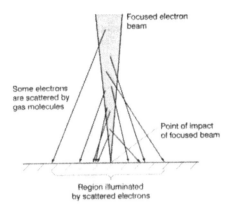

Focused electron beam

Some electrons are scattered by gas molecules

Point of impact of focused beam

Region illuminated by scattered electrons

Figure 5.10. Sketch showing how some electrons are scattered by the gas in a low-pressure environment, while others reach the sample as a focused probe.

resolution image. All the electrons, of course, also potentially generate X-rays. Unfortunately, there is no equivalent to the background subtraction of the electron image. It is not, in general, possible to identify what component of the analysis results from the main probe, and what is generated by the scattered electrons. *Figure 5.11* shows spectra taken in an ESEM from a thin iron disc placed on a standard Al sample stub. The spectra were obtained from a point about 0.1 mm from the edge of the disc. The solid spectrum was obtained with a very low pressure (<0.1 torr) in the chamber, and very little, if any, trace of Al is seen. The dotted curve was the spectrum obtained after increasing the pressure in the chamber to 4 torr. (The spectra were normalized so that the backgrounds overlapped exactly.) A strong peak from Al is present in this latter spectrum, demonstrating that the primary electrons are being scattered to points at least 0.1 mm away from the nominal beam position.

The scattering effect can be mitigated by operating the microscope at as low a pressure as is compatible with controlling the charging. In addition, using a very light gas (such as helium) rather than the typical water vapor, can lead to less scattering, though possibly with reduced image quality. In the ESEM, use of the so-called 'X-ray bullet' can also reduce the scattering by reducing the path length of the electrons in the gas. None of these precautions was taken in preparing the data for *Figure 5.11*, but if a gas is present, some scattering will always occur and will result in degraded X-ray analytical precision.

As can be seen from *Figure 5.11*, and as would be expected from an understanding of the problem, the contribution of scattered electrons to the X-ray signal is reduced by reducing the gas pressure. Unfortunately, this can lead to charging of the sample, with disastrous consequences for the microanalysis. The effect is made more problematic because it is insidious – unless the operator looks for the effect, it is easy to miss. This second difficulty arises because the ESEM and VP-SEM do not *eliminate* charging on the surface, they only *control* it. In many operating conditions, the supply of positive ions near the sample surface is adequate to allow charge balance when the surface is only very slightly charged. However, in some circumstances, which particularly include low-pressure operation,

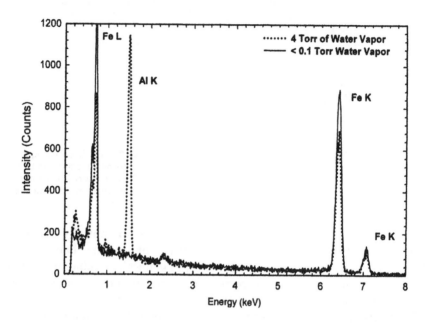

Figure 5.11. Spectra obtained at 20 kV in an ESEM with the electron probe 0.1 mm away from the edge of an Fe disc 3 mm in diameter on an Al substrate, at low pressure (solid curve) and with a pressure of 4 torr of water vapor (dots). Other experimental conditions were the same for the two acquisitions. The large Al signal in the dotted spectrum arises from electrons scattered by the gas.

the supply of positive ions is very limited. The surface charges to many hundreds of volts, or even kilovolts, before it attracts an adequate supply of ions to maintain a balance with the charge brought in by the incident beam. This has the effect of decelerating the incident electrons. Thus the beam energy arriving at the sample is lower (sometimes very much lower) than the voltage setting of the SEM. As we have seen, the beam voltage has major effects on the production of X-rays in the sample, so any attempt at semi-quantitative analysis will give possibly wildly wrong answers. Despite this, the effect of the charging on the image may be quite subtle, and even an experienced operator may not notice the significance of it. Checking the apparent beam voltage by looking for the Duane–Hunt limit, as described earlier in this chapter, will immediately show whether charging is taking place.

We should note here that the effect is not limited to the VP-SEM and ESEM. Even when a conductive coat is applied to the sample to bleed away surface charge, it is possible, in many insulators, for charge to accumulate in the lattice below the surface. This has precisely the same effect in decelerating the beam, but may not be so obvious in the Duane–Hunt limit. Since the surface is at ground potential the electrons actually arrive there with their original energy. Only after they penetrate the surface do they experience the deceleration, so some bremsstrahlung X-rays are generated up to the energy of the beam. The shape of the continuum is only altered in a subtle way, but the effect on the microanalysis can still be profound.

5.6 Inhomogeneous samples

In the context of this chapter, we consider all samples that do not have a constant composition over the entire volume affected, directly or indirectly, by the incident electron beam and its products, to be 'inhomogeneous'. A consequence of this definition is that, in such samples, even the 'semi-quantitative' analysis described in Section 5.4 is subject at best to more uncertainties, and may often not be possible.

While analysis of inhomogeneous samples is a very different undertaking from that discussed so far, often much useful information can be obtained, especially if the geometry of the sample is well defined. We shall discuss one such case in a moment. First, let us consider cases in which the microanalysis is obviously difficult.

As an example, consider a two-phase material in which one, or both, of the phases exist in forms with dimensions equal to, or smaller than, the interaction volume of the electron probe. The smaller the dimensions of the phase, the harder it becomes to extract any useful data from the analysis. It is often helpful in such cases to consider reducing the electron beam voltage, as this reduces the interaction volume. A difficulty, of course, is that the excitation of the more energetic lines in the X-ray spectrum is also reduced or eliminated. An illustration of this effect will be given in Chapter 7, where we show X-ray maps obtained from a Pb–Sn alloy (i.e. solder) at different beam voltages.

There are other drawbacks to this technique. As the beam energy is reduced, so the gun brightness, and hence the electron current, decreases, thus reducing still further the number of X-rays produced. As we have observed, often the generation of higher-energy X-ray lines will be completely absent, and only very low-energy lines will be excited. However, the energy resolution of the detector may be insufficient to resolve them. It is for problems like this that the microcalorimeter detector, which we discussed in Section 3.5.2, would be ideal.

Often, applying knowledge of the production and detection of X-rays can lead to informative conclusions about the sample. *Figure 5.12* shows a spectrum that includes Ni and a very small amount of Cu. It was obtained with a beam energy of 30 keV. Significantly, if one examines critically the ratios between the Cu K and L lines, and the Ni K and L lines, one sees that the K/L ratio is far higher for the Ni than it is for the Cu. In fact, if one is used to thin foil analysis in the TEM (the subject of the next chapter), one might think that this ratio for the Cu is more typical of a thin film. What the analysis is telling us is that we have a thin film of Cu on the surface of the Ni. We can actually do better than this – we can (approximately) measure the thickness of the film!

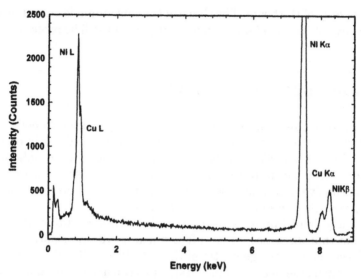

Figure 5.12. EDX spectrum obtained at 30 keV in the SEM, showing Ni and Cu. The ratio of the Ni K and L peaks is typical of solid samples; the equivalent ratio for Cu is typical of thin films. The sample was a Ni ball with a thin evaporated layer of Cu on the surface.

To achieve this feat, we need the help of modelling software. Given the confidence in models for the generation and absorption of X-rays, which follows from their success at interpreting X-ray spectra from homogeneous samples, it is only a small step to apply them to other specimen geometries. The thin film on a substrate is one of the simpler of these situations. One can either use analytic expressions that essentially assume a specimen geometry and composition, and compute the X-ray generation, absorption and fluorescence to predict the acquired spectrum, or one can use a Monte Carlo calculation. In either case, by adjusting the modelled thickness of the Cu film on the Ni surface, until the predicted X-ray spectrum matches the experimental one, it is possible to make an estimate of the actual film thickness. To confirm the result, the experiment can be repeated at one or more different beam voltages. If each experiment gives the same film thickness, then the result is confirmed with some confidence. If the result varies significantly (and especially if the variation is consistent at different beam voltages), then one may suspect that there is a problem with the interpretation – perhaps some Cu is in solution in the Ni, and some on the surface. Further investigation would be in order at this point.

Returning to *Figure 5.12*, the sample was actually solid Ni, with a random thickness of Cu evaporated onto the surface. The simulation was once again performed by Electron Flight Simulator. Comparing the heights of the L lines, as in the illustration, the best fit to the measured spectrum is obtained by modelling a film 120 nm thick. There are short-comings with the method, arising from imperfect knowledge of the various physical parameters involved in the interaction, and a series of different experiments, at different beam voltages and modelling both the K lines and L lines actually give values for the thickness ranging from 60 to 160 nm. For critical situations, the user, naturally, would test any modelling software with carefully prepared samples of known characteristics before trusting any results obtained from unknown samples. With care, ingenuity and patience, it is possible to derive information about several layers on top of each other, although the applicability will depend upon the exact details of the sample (chemistry of the layers, their thickness, etc.). Data can be obtained to a depth of 1 μm or more in suitable samples.

Other geometries are amenable, to a greater or lesser extent, to similar analysis. Another example would be spherical particles, either in isolation or embedded in a matrix. Obviously, the more complex the situation, and the less precisely it is understood, the more the uncertainty in the interpretation of the spectra.

5.7 Concluding remarks

It has, obviously, not been our goal in this chapter to make the reader an expert in microanalysis in the SEM. At least one two-volume work has been dedicated to that task, as well as numerous other complete books. Active research continues in the techniques of quantitative analysis, for example in methods to obtain more precise analyses from rough surfaces, and in methods to achieve better precision in the analysis of light elements.

We hope we have given enough explanation to point out why X-ray analysis in the SEM and microprobe is such a complex subject, enabling the person planning to make measurements to get a feel for what compromises are available between training, experience, effort at making measurements and the quality of the results. While it is often true that a little knowledge is a bad thing, it is most certainly true that a modest understanding of X-ray analysis in the SEM can lead to the acquisition of results, which, while possibly limited in some ways, are nevertheless extremely useful, because the limitations are understood and accounted for in the interpretation.

6 X-ray microanalysis in the transmission electron microscope

6.1 Introduction

Performing scanning electron microscopy on a sample is generally a relatively undemanding task. Only one surface of the sample must be accessible, so there is no major constraint on the sample size. However, as we saw in Chapter 5, the spatial resolution of microanalysis is limited, both in the SEM and the electron microprobe, not by the size of the electron probe but by the volume of the sample into which the probe diffuses. We also saw the difficulties associated with performing quantitative analysis on anything but carefully prepared polished surfaces.

While microanalysis in the TEM requires very complex sample preparation, and so could not be described as addressing the second difficulty mentioned above, it does provide a method of improving the spatial resolution by at least two orders of magnitude, without sacrificing precision or sensitivity. While the atom probe can claim to be the instrument with the highest spatial resolution (it analyses a sample atom-by-atom), the purpose-built analytical TEM can, at least in principle, analyse a 1-nm diameter particle with enough sensitivity to be limited by the statistics of the number of atoms in the particle. The same instrument, at the turn of a knob, can generate an image covering about 0.05 mm of the sample. This flexibility makes it an extremely powerful tool for the materials scientist.

A simple description of X-ray microanalysis of thin films in the TEM might, indeed, be presented as follows: 'A focused beam of electrons falls on a thin sample, generating characteristic X-rays. The intensity of each characteristic peak in the spectrum is proportional to the concentration of the element in the sample, the proportionality constant depending on the element, the beam energy and the detector, but not on the physical state of the sample, and the spatial resolution is determined by the diameter of the electron probe and the thickness of the sample.' While this statement does provide significant insight into the technique, and may actually suffice to describe simple analytical problems, the reality is far more complex in detail, as we shall see. In the organization of this chapter, we shall start from this simple statement, and consider the issues that must be borne in mind in a demanding analytical situation.

We will assume that the reader will be using a microscope in which the objective lens is designed for the formation of fine electron probes. All TEM/STEM and dedicated STEM instruments are in this category, and many other modern instruments also have the capability, even though they may not have the ability to form a scanned image of the sample. Some TEMs, though, have an electron-optical configuration that precludes the formation of optimized probes. If these instruments are fitted with X-ray detectors, microanalysis will still be possible, but not with the sensitivity and spatial resolution we suggest here.

6.2 Principles of quantitative analysis in the TEM

We remember from the preceding chapters that the sensitivity of X-ray detectors to X-rays of different energies can vary significantly; in particular, the sensitivity to very soft X-rays can be very low. Particularly this is the case with detectors fitted with beryllium windows (mainly older detectors). Unfortunately, the light elements only produce soft X-rays (the emission from hydrogen and helium is considered to be UV, as it is so soft). Many samples (polymers, almost all biological specimens, oxides, etc.) contain significant quantities of these 'difficult' elements; special techniques, which we shall discuss briefly in a moment, have been developed to perform quantitative analysis of such specimens. For now, we will consider only situations in which X-rays from all the elements in a sample are measurable.

6.2.1 Cliff–Lorimer method

Most quantitative thin film analysis in the TEM makes use of the Cliff–Lorimer equation:

$$\frac{I_A}{I_B} = \frac{C_A}{C_B} \cdot k_{AB} \tag{6.1}$$

where I_A and I_B are respectively the intensities of the characteristic peaks from elements A and B, C_A and C_B are the concentrations of the elements in the sample, and k_{AB} is a proportionality 'constant', whose value depends upon a number of factors. This equation was first published in 1975, and, following the conventions of metallurgy, the concentrations were expressed in weight fraction. This has remained the standard practice of most analysts, though of course the concentration could equally well be expressed in atomic fraction (with a different numerical value of k_{AB}). The factor k_{AB} has become universally known as the 'Cliff–Lorimer k-factor'.

It will be helpful if we look more closely at the derivation of the Cliff–Lorimer equation. We remember from Chapter 2 that the generation of a characteristic X-ray is a two-step process; first, an atom must be excited by an electron-induced ionization event, then the excited atom must decay to the ground state by emitting an X-ray. The ionization event is characterized by a cross-section Q, which depends upon the incident electron energy, and the decay is characterized by a fluorescence yield ω. It is usually also necessary to remember to include in computations the partition fraction s, because typically only a single member of a family of X-ray lines will be used for quantitative analysis. If we have a very thin sample made of elements A and B as above, then the number of X-rays generated per second I'_A of element A can be written as:

$$I'_A = \frac{N_o}{A_A} \cdot \frac{i_p}{e} \cdot \rho \cdot t \cdot C_A \cdot Q_A \cdot \omega_A \cdot s_A \qquad (6.2)$$

where N_o is Avogadro's number, A_A is the atomic weight of element A, i_p is the electron probe current e is the electronic charge, and ρ and t are, respectively, the density and the thickness of the sample. Since the emission of the X-rays is isotropic, the number detected I_A will be related to I'_A by

$$I_A = I'_A \cdot \varepsilon_A \qquad (6.3)$$

where the detector efficiency ε_A is shown as a function of the element because of the energy-dependence of the detector response. A similar equation can be written for I_B. Dividing one by the other results in the following expression:

$$\frac{I_A}{I_B} = \frac{A_B}{A_A} \cdot \frac{Q_A \cdot \omega_A \cdot \varepsilon_A \cdot s_A}{Q_B \cdot \omega_B \cdot \varepsilon_B \cdot s_B} \cdot \frac{C_A}{C_B} \qquad (6.4)$$

The Qs are a function of the beam voltage (though, for the electron energies typically used in the transmission microscopy their ratio is a relatively weak function of the voltage), the ωs and ss are constants for a particular transition, the εs are, within some limits, constant for a particular X-ray detector, and the As are, of course, constant, so, for a particular electron beam voltage in a particular electron microscope, this expression can be seen to be equivalent to Equation 6.1.

From the preceding discussion it can be seen that the Cliff–Lorimer k-factor is not strictly a constant, having a weak dependence on the beam voltage and a significant dependence on the detector efficiency. For the sake of completeness, it should be mentioned that the caveat we introduced earlier, that the sample be 'very thin', allows us to ignore the absorption of X-rays within the sample, and the loss of energy of the electrons as they propagate through the sample, with the resultant change in ionization cross-section (the $\phi(\rho,z)$ effect important in microprobe analysis). Because of the dependence on the detector efficiency, some authors have written the Cliff–Lorimer equation in the form

$$\frac{I_A}{I_B} = k_{AB} \frac{C_A}{C_B} \cdot \frac{\varepsilon_A}{\varepsilon_B}$$ (6.5)

in an effort to define a more universal k-value.

Unfortunately, even on a specific instrument, the detector efficiency cannot be assumed to be constant. As we discussed in Chapter 3, over time, the crystal may acquire a layer of ice, which will effectively absorb soft X-rays. If quantitative analysis of light elements is to be undertaken, it is essential to monitor the build-up of this ice (or other contamination) by routine analysis of a standard sample of NiO thin film or in whatever other way the operator chooses. Fortunately, except in severe cases, these changes in sensitivity affect only the detection of soft X-rays – those whose energies are below about 2 keV. For more energetic X-rays, at least up to about 20 keV, all detectors have a detection probability (i.e. the probability of recording the arrival of an X-ray that does, in fact, reach the detector) approaching unity.

We have seen how the k-factor relates the observed X-ray intensities to the elemental concentrations in the sample. How are these factors determined?

If the parameters in Equation 6.4 are all known, then, of course, the k-factor can be calculated. We discussed in Chapter 2, though, that while expressions exist for modelling the ionization cross-sections, they are not very precise, especially for ionization of shells other than the K shell. The fluorescence yield is likewise subject to some uncertainty. As we saw in Chapter 3, the detector efficiency can vary somewhat from detector to detector, and as a function of time, especially for the light elements. Hence, while it is possible to use theoretical or published values of the parameters in Equation 6.4 to calculate the k-factor, the result should not be considered precise, especially when comparing X-ray lines of different series. As a general rule, computed k-factors are most trustworthy for K-lines, and especially for lines of similar energy.

The alternative approach is to measure the k-factor by acquiring a spectrum from a sample of known composition. The analyst must be careful to account for issues such as absorption and fluorescence (which will be discussed in Section 6.3), but if this is done, then this method provides probably the most precise way of obtaining the k-factor. The principal difficulty, oddly enough, is in the provision of a suitable sample, which is sufficiently homogeneous, on both a coarse and a fine scale, to allow the analyst to be certain of the composition of the areas selected for the standardization measurements.

Sometimes the experiment permits some feature or phase of the sample to serve as a calibration standard. This may especially be the case if the important property being determined is the difference in composition from one area to another, rather than the absolute composition of each area. An example of this may be an investigation of grain boundary segregation, when the composition of the grain matrix might be assumed to equal the known overall composition of the sample (measurement of interface segregation will be discussed later in this chapter).

It is clear, of course, that if the k-factor for two elements, let us say A and B, is required, but only the relative k-factors of each of the elements to a third element, let us say X, are known, then the simple relation $k_{AB}=k_{AX}/k_{BX}$ holds. Some of the early research on k-factors was performed on silicate minerals, for the simple, and very important, reason that they provided a well-characterized and trustworthy set of standards. The k-factors were naturally computed relative to the common element, silicon. As a result, it became for a time conventional to use silicon as the third element 'X' for specifying all k-factors. There is, of course, no fundamental reason why this must be done, and later authors have argued that there are significant disadvantages to the use of silicon for this purpose, and have instead used Fe as the reference element. Providing the details of the standardization measurements are clearly understood, there is no significance in the choice, and the analyst is free to adopt any standardization method that suits the convenience and meets the needs of the investigation.

6.2.2 Hall method

We mentioned in the introduction to this section that difficulties arise in quantitative analysis when one or more of the elements present does not generate observable, or at least useful, X-rays. If a detector with a beryllium window is in use, then such samples would include all ceramics (oxides, carbides, nitrides, etc.) as well as almost all samples of biological origin. Even when a light-element detector is in use, the difficulties and uncertainties involved in quantifying soft X-rays can lead to unacceptable errors for many of these samples.

In some cases (many oxides, for example), it is satisfactory to assume the concentration of the element from stoichiometry. The assumed composition can then be used in computing an absorption correction (if required – see the following section). In other cases, though, an absolute measurement of the composition must be made without any foreknowledge about the sample. Many measurements on biological systems would fall into this category.

If all that is required is the ratio of one measurable element to another (K to Ca, for example), then the procedures of the preceding sub-section could be applied. If the absolute concentration of one of the elements was known, then the absolute concentration of the other would be immediately derived. More problematic, though, is the general case when the absolute concentration of no element is known.

The Hall method of microanalysis, originally proposed by Marshall and Hall in 1966, and revisited and revised by Hall and co-workers, and others, in a number of papers since then, is a way of deriving absolute concentrations of heavy elements in the presence of a very light matrix. The method compares the intensity of the characteristic peaks of the unknown elements with the intensity of the bremsstrahlung background generated by the entire sample.

In Chapter 2 we discussed the generation of bremsstrahlung and characteristic X-rays. While we did not go into detail, we mentioned that both processes are predictable, and that while the bremsstrahlung shape is, to a first approximation at least, independent of the sample, the intensity of the background is a strong function of the mean atomic number of the sample (a linear function in Kramer's relationship, Equation 2.1, but a more complex function in more recent background models). Provided the mean atomic number of the sample can be assumed (from some independent knowledge, for example), then the intensity of the bremsstrahlung leads to a knowledge of the mass–thickness of the sample. The characteristic intensity from the heavy element leads to a knowledge of the effective mass–thickness of that element. The ratio of the two numbers leads directly to the absolute concentration.

As with so many techniques in science, while the description of the technique is rather simple, its effective implementation is quite the contrary. One problem for the casual user arises from the policies of most EDX vendors. It is usual for sellers of EDX systems to include in the quoted price a choice of one quantitative analysis package, the options being SEM, materials TEM or biological TEM. We have anecdotal evidence that tells us that very few purchasers select the biological package. Hence the typical user, coming to an average TEM facility, is unlikely to find biological quantitative software available.

Other, more severe problems plague the analyst. Since, in most cases, the concentrations of the elements being sought are quite low, extended counting times are required. This places extreme stability constraints on the sample. Any loss of mass due to beam damage, for example, will invalidate the measurement, as will any build-up of contamination during the analysis. The method cannot be applied, of course, to biological samples that have been fixed, mounted and sectioned. Even the thickness of a carbon support film (if used) must be allowed for.

We have seen in earlier chapters how stray X-rays may be generated, and subsequently recorded by the X-ray detector. It has been commonly observed that peak to background ratios measured from known samples differ, not only from theoretically predicted values, but also from one instrument to another, even though the nominal analytical configuration may be the same. These differences are attributable to the stray X-rays. For successful application of the Hall method, the stray X-ray intensity must either be known to be insignificant, or a means must be available to allow for it.

As was shown in a published review by Fiori *et al.* (1986), even such fundamental details as the appropriate model to use for the cross-sections are not firmly established. A user of commercial software should investigate carefully the models upon which the software was based, before relying on its output.

The Hall method of quantification of solute concentrations in light materials has been used very successfully in a few laboratories, where all these problems have been carefully researched, and procedures developed to overcome them. For the casual user, though, the obstacles to performing reliable analysis are so high that measurements are rarely attempted.

6.3 Absorption, fluorescence and other sources of error

The thin-film Cliff–Lorimer method of quantification we have discussed depends on the assumption that the measured X-ray signal is accurately and predictably related to the generated X-rays, taking into account such 'constants' as the change in sensitivity of the X-ray detector with energy. We must, though, also consider processes by which the generated X-ray spectrum may be altered, in less predictable ways, before it is detected and recorded.

As we saw in Equation 6.3, the X-ray count rate depends on the sample thickness. If the sample is too thin, the count rate goes down, and the precision of the analysis degrades. On the other hand, if the sample gets too thick, the electron beam will broaden out as it propagates through the foil, and effects such as X-ray absorption and fluorescence will degrade the analysis. Beam broadening affects the spatial resolution of the experiment; we will delay discussion of it to Section 6.5. Here we will discuss absorption and fluorescence, which can alter the analytical precision of the measurement. We will also need to consider the effect of electrons, other than those in the primary beam, striking the sample.

6.3.1 Self-absorption of X-rays in the sample

In Chapter 5 we saw how X-rays generated at different depths in the solid sample have to travel through different distances of material to reach the X-ray detector, and how the associated probability of their being absorbed complicates quantitative analysis. The far shorter absorption paths in the thin sample reduce, but do not eliminate, the possibility of absorption of the X-rays, and this still must be taken into account if the highest precision analysis is sought. Fluorescence within the sample is likewise much less significant than in SEM analysis, but must be considered, and in some cases allowed for. On the other hand, it has been shown that in virtually all cases, the change in energy of the electron beam as it propagates through the foil has an insignificant effect on the X-ray production, and can therefore be ignored.

It is quite easy to model the absorption, provided the geometry is known. It is readily shown that, for the geometry of *Figure 6.1*, and using the nomenclature of that illustration,

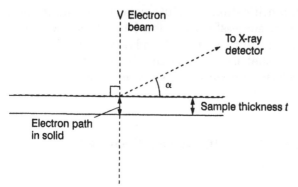

Figure 6.1. Sketch of the ideal geometry of the sample in TEM X-ray analysis.

$$R_{A,B} = R_{A,B,o} \cdot \frac{\left.\dfrac{\mu}{\rho}\right|_{Spec}^{A}}{\left.\dfrac{\mu}{\rho}\right|_{Spec}^{B}} \cdot \frac{\left[1 - \exp-\left\{\left.\dfrac{\mu}{\rho}\right|_{Spec}^{B} \cdot \mathrm{cosec}\alpha(\rho t)\right\}\right]}{\left[1 - \exp-\left\{\left.\dfrac{\mu}{\rho}\right|_{Spec}^{A} \cdot \mathrm{cosec}\alpha(\rho t)\right\}\right]} \qquad (6.6)$$

where $R_{A,B,o}$ is the ratio between the generated X-ray intensities of elements A and B, $R_{A,B}$ is the emitted ratio, $\left.\dfrac{\mu}{\rho}\right|_{Spec}^{Ele}$ is the mass absorption coefficient of the sample for the particular energy of X-rays under consideration, and ρ is the sample density. A similar, and only slightly more complex, equation applies in the case of the sample tilted with respect to the beam.

Since successful electron microprobe analysis requires accurate knowledge of the mass absorption coefficients, an extensive literature exists on the topic, as we described in Chapter 5. Hence these equations may be used as the basis for a correction for self-absorption. It is important to understand, though, that the correction only applies in the case of a homogeneous, parallel-sided foil of known tilt and thickness. Unfortunately, most samples are heterogeneous and of unknown geometry, as for example, in *Figure 6.2*. Even the measurement of the sample thickness is a major challenge. Hence, while in some specific cases thickness corrections can be applied, in most work the practical significance of Equation 6.6 is that it gives an estimate of the error introduced by ignoring absorption (or, conversely, indicates when it is legitimate to ignore it).

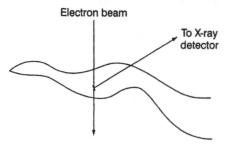

Figure 6.2. Sketch of the more usual unpredictable sample geometry.

An alternative approach to correcting for the self-absorption is to use the shape of the bremsstrahlung continuum. The continuum X-rays are generated throughout the sample and are subject to exactly the same absorption path as the characteristic X-rays. Hence, if the continuum shape is known or can be reliably modelled, a comparison between the prediction and the actually recorded spectrum immediately leads to the absorption at any X-ray energy. The method only works, however, if the microscope is 'clean', in the sense that essentially no X-rays are recorded other than those directly resulting from the interaction of the electron beam with the sample. This is a very difficult condition to satisfy. This method of self-absorption correction is more general than the analytic approach discussed above, in that neither the local specimen geometry nor the sample thickness need be known; however, while it may give a better approximation to the correct analysis than would the raw data, the necessity of applying any correction should be avoided, or at least minimized, as far as possible. Interestingly, as the data required for computing the correction are stored with the spectrum, an absorption correction can be made 'after the fact'. Incidentally, by making reasonable assumptions about the sample tilt, an approximation of the sample thickness can be obtained by this method with at least as much precision as with any other readily available technique, except for the use of electron energy-loss spectroscopy, which is applicable only to relatively thin samples. An example of this application is shown in *Figure 6.3*, which shows the spectrum obtained from a sample of $BaTiO_4$; the model of the spectrum generated by DTSA is overlaid. The model assumed an ice thickness of 0.9 μm (derived from other measurements on very thin samples), and a sample thickness of 500 nm. The small Cu signal – not included in the model – arose from a Cu support ring round the sample, and the silicon was a component of the contamination, which was severe on this sample. The ratio of peak to bremsstrahlung background was only modelled correctly when allowance was made for the contamination layer – which, of course, contributes to the bremsstrahlung. The remaining differences between the model and the observed spectrum are interesting – the peak in the observed spectrum just above the O peak is the sum peak of one O and one C X-ray; the disagreement between the model and the observed spectrum in the region of the Ba M peak (just higher in energy than the sum peak just mentioned) is due to a sum peak of two O X-rays, and the small excess in the background in the spectral region below the Ba and Ti peaks is due to degraded events. The relative sizes of the O and the Ba and Ti peaks (which overlap each other) agree in the model and observed spectrum, although at the scale the illustration is plotted this is not visible. These ratios are significantly different for modelled sample thicknesses of 400 or 600 nm. This method of sample thickness determination is not very precise, because the main effect of the sample thickness is observed in the low-energy region of the spectrum, where other spurious processes (sum peaks, degraded events or contamination layers, for example) can also have an influence. However, it can certainly usefully increase the analyst's knowledge of the sample.

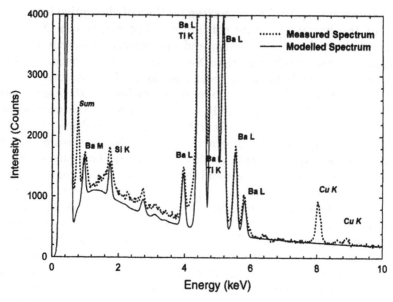

Figure 6.3. Spectrum of barium titanate, with a model showing an excellent agreement for a sample thickness of 500 nm. This is described further in Section 6.3.1.

It should be emphasized that the mass absorption coefficients used in Equation 6.6 must take into account all the elements present in the sample – even if they do not generate visible X-ray peaks. Light elements such as C, nitrogen and O, which are not seen with a beryllium-windowed detector, can still absorb other X-rays significantly, and degrade the precision of the analysis.

6.3.2 Fluorescence

X-rays generated from within the sample travel not only towards the X-ray detector, but in all directions; they will finally interact with some part of the sample remote from the point of impact of the beam, the sample holder, the lens pole-pieces or some other part of the microscope. In all cases, the X-ray can cause fluorescence of characteristic X-rays of some lower energy. It is possible that these X-rays can be emitted towards the X-ray detector, and be recorded as part of the spectrum from the sample.

The first line of defence against these fluoresced X-rays is the collimation of the detector. By limiting the field of view of the detector as far as possible to the region of the sample, the fluoresced X-rays originating from remote areas can be prevented from entering the X-ray detector and being included in the spectrum. It is impossible, though, to eliminate every spurious X-ray. Unfortunately, the conditions needed for high-sensitivity, high-resolution analysis (to be discussed in the next section) conflict with the need for highly efficient collimation. X-ray fluorescence will always contribute to a thin-film X-ray spectrum.

The microscopist (or person responsible for the long-term care of the microscope) should, of course, initially characterize the instrument by obtaining spectra for long counting times and high probe currents from a variety of pure samples, including heavier materials. This will allow spectra to be examined for the presence of any systematic lines which could arise from materials within the microscope, including the pole-pieces and the specimen holder (the measurements would, of course, be repeated for all available sample holders). While it would be difficult to be quantitative, the analyst would thus know what lines, when seen at a very low level, may be due to fluorescence from the instrument. We note that various 'test' samples have been proposed for investigating fluorescence effects in TEMs. For the average user, on a day-to-day basis, these samples are probably 'overkill' (though they would provide the required information). The main application of such samples is in the evaluation of new specimen/detector configurations implemented by manufacturers or ambitious microscope owners.

If possible, an experiment should be arranged so that fluorescence can be identified and hence accounted for. As an example, small particles can be analysed while supported on a thin carbon film on a Cu grid. The majority of the fluorescence will be from the Cu; assuming Cu is not in the sample, the Cu can be ignored (if Cu is of interest in the sample, a different choice of support grid would be made – an extensive selection is available commercially).

In many cases, though, the principal source of fluoresced radiation will be the sample itself. This is particularly insidious because all the detected X-rays will be from elements known to be in the sample. The difficulty that is created arises because the probability of exciting X-rays by self-fluorescence from the different elements is widely different from the probability of exciting them by X-ray bombardment. In the case of the homogeneous parallel-sided thin foil, as illustrated in *Figure 6.1*, the process can be modelled, and an analytic expression for a correction can be derived. We will not describe the correction theory here, referring readers to the texts identified in the bibliography. In specific cases, it does work – at least, in the sense that the 'corrected' analysis can be shown to be closer to the expected value than the 'uncorrected' analysis. Fluorescence, though, is far more sensitive to the sample geometry at some distance from the analysis point than is absorption; *Figure 6.4* shows one example.

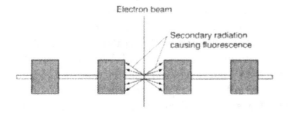

Figure 6.4. Sketch showing how fluorescence can be generated in a heterogeneous sample.

It is sometimes possible to deduce, from a knowledge of the experiment, that the fluorescence correction is likely to be small. For example, a lower-energy X-ray line cannot excite a higher-energy one. Such a case would be a small concentration of Ni in Fe. On the other hand, if the major element were Ni, then its X-rays could certainly fluoresce the Fe.

Zaluzec (1984) has examined the problem of applying fluorescence corrections, from the point of view of the experimenter. He derived some guidelines, the chief of which is that if the atomic number of the fluoresced element and the emitter of the fluorescing radiation differ by more than two, then fluorescence is unlikely to be a significant problem. It must be understood, though, that his work was assuming a homogeneous sample of known geometry. As we have said before, few samples actually meet that criterion. Unfortunately, in the general case, the analyst will have to be content with the understanding that fluorescence may be limiting the precision of the analysis.

6.3.3 *Excitation by electrons*

Here we are not concerned with the excitation by the primary beam of electrons; this is generating the desired signal. Rather, we are concerned by excitation of the sample by bombardment of points remote from the position of interest. Such electron bombardment can arise from stray electrons present in the microscope column or from electrons scattered from the sample itself. The two can be differentiated by passing the beam through a small hole in the sample and recording an X-ray spectrum. If stray radiation is present a significant spectrum will be seen (in this text we will shirk the responsibility of defining 'significant' in this context); if only a few counts per second are recorded then the electron column is 'clean'. The spectrum obtained in these circumstances is called the 'hole count' for obvious reasons. The hole count is strongly dependent on the design of the electron column and the choice of aperture styles, and only to a limited extent on the operating choices of the operator. If the hole count is significant, a first approximation of a correction may be made by recording the hole count under identical microscope conditions as are used to obtain the spectrum from the sample, and subtracting. This, of course, degrades the noise level in the spectrum (as already mentioned, statistically, subtraction has exactly the same effect as addition), and care must be taken that the conditions are as nearly as possible exactly the same for all spectra (including the emission current from the gun).

Figure 6.5 shows ways in which electrons scattered from the sample can generate X-rays. The intensity of the spurious signal from the sample itself is a strong function of the sample tilt. This can be illustrated by examining a sample – not containing Cu – supported on a Cu grid. With the sample horizontal, record an X-ray spectrum and note the ratio between the signal from the sample and the Cu. Then tilt the sample – in any direction – and repeat the measurement. The Cu signal will be seen to have increased. *Figure 6.6* shows an example of this experiment, in this case, cerium oxide

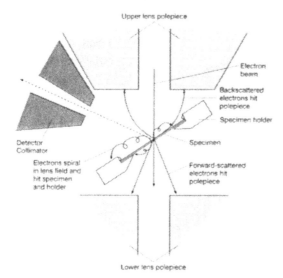

Figure 6.5. Sketch showing how stray radiation (scattered electrons and X-rays) can interact with the sample and other parts of the microscope structure to generate spurious X-rays.

particles (doped, in this case, with some gold) on a carbon film/Cu grid substrate. The substantial increase in the Cu signal in the tilted case is clear. Because cerium is a relatively heavy element it scatters electrons efficiently. If the same experiment was performed with, say, Al_2O_3 particles, the Cu signal would be much lower. In our microscope, very few X-rays are recorded from the sample holder, the pole-pieces or other parts of the system, but this is not the case for all instruments, especially older ones.

Degradation of the precision of analysis by this mechanism is not predictable, and therefore not correctable. The significance will vary from analysis to analysis, and must be borne in mind by the analyst in judging the overall precision of the measurement.

6.3.4 Excitation by stray X-rays

By 'stray' X-rays, we mean, in this section, X-rays generated in the microscope column as a result of the electron beam striking parts of the microscope structure. The most significant, but not the only one, of these, perhaps, is the beam-limiting aperture. The aperture is usually made of a moderately heavy material (typically either platinum or Mo), and as a result, not only are the characteristic X-rays of the sample material excited, but also an intense bremsstrahlung continuum, extending in energy up to the beam energy, is present. In modern, so-called intermediate-voltage instruments, this limit may be 300 keV or more. These high-energy X-rays are able to penetrate the aperture thickness, and, unless prevented by the design of the microscope, will strike the sample in an unfocussed spot, leading to the generation of characteristic X-rays, which will be recorded by the detector. The effect will be similar to that described above as the 'hole count', generated by stray electrons in the

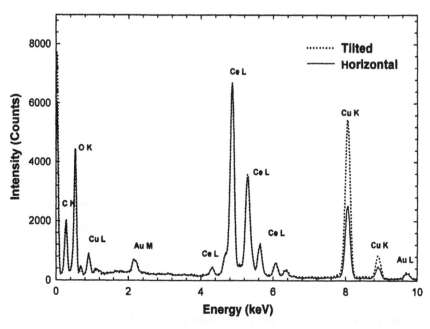

Figure 6.6. Spectra obtained at 250keV of a cerium oxide particle supported on a C film and Cu grid, horizontal (solid line) and tilted 20° (dots). The change in the spurious Cu signal is obvious. In this system the Ce, being a relatively heavy element, scatters the electrons efficiently, leading to more excitation of the Cu than would be observed in, say, a spectrum from Al_2O_3 particles on a similar grid.

column, except that the ratios of the different elements in the spectrum will probably be quite different.

In general, the same strategies mitigate both electron-excited and X-ray-excited hole counts. These include locating the beam-limiting aperture as far from the sample as other design constraints allow, using a compound structure for the aperture, and using other, non-limiting apertures between the beam-limiting aperture and the sample, to block the stray radiation. *Figure 6.7* shows spectra acquired from a hole in the carbon film of the same specimen, and otherwise in the same conditions, as *Figure 6.6*, with and without the selected area aperture in place. Again, the difference is clear. *Figures 6.6* and *6.7* are shown at different scales – even without the aperture, the hole count is actually insignificant with respect to the specimen spectrum, demonstrating that this particular microscope is very 'clean' for the purposes of X-ray analysis.

6.3.5 *Precision of quantitative analysis*

It will be apparent to the reader that there are a number of conflicting issues when attempting to optimize an analysis in the TEM. Firstly, the need for a large number of counts means, as we have seen, that the product

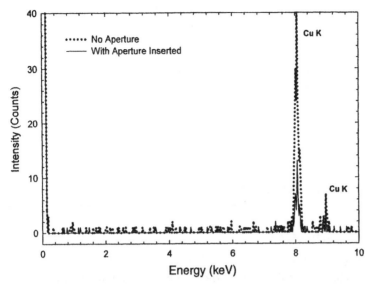

Figure 6.7. Spectra taken at 250 keV from a hole in the film of the same sample as *Figure 6.6*, showing the difference between the spectra acquired with a selected area aperture in place (solid curve) and without (dots). Other details of the acquisition were the same for both spectra. It is clear that the aperture is effective in limiting the stray radiation that reaches the sample from remote parts of the electron column.

of the sample thickness and the probe current be kept relatively high. We discuss later the mechanics of optimizing the electron probe. For now, we will observe that the typical user, when faced with the need to acquire counts at a higher count-rate will generally move to a thicker region. Unfortunately this may well create problems with self-absorption (depending on the analysis). The correct approach would be to increase the beam current by increasing the probe size. In general a probe optimized for microanalytical precision will result in an image – at high magnification at least – that does not appear sharp (which means that in order to take a sharp photograph of the sample, the probe will have to be readjusted).

If statistical precision was the only limit in quantitative analysis, we have seen in Chapter 3 that we would be able to analyse to within ± 0.1% or better. As we have seen though, there are other factors. We have already discussed absorption, which can easily introduce a 1% error, fluorescence (which can often be negligible, but in other cases introduce errors of the order of a few percent), the precision of the knowledge of the k-factors and stray signals. We must also be concerned that the thin sample is representative of the bulk. The sample can be changed during the thinning process. For example, if an area 40 nm thick (which would appear moderately thin in the microscope, but is easily achievable) has a single monolayer of a trace element concentrated on the surfaces, the result will appear to be a concentration of 1% of the trace element in the analysis. Depending on the preparation method, such a layer could easily be present. Likewise, if radiation damage caused by the energetic electrons causes chemical changes in the sample, then the acquired spectrum will not represent the original composition.

Most of these factors will vary from analysis to analysis. Hence, in one experiment, the precision may only be ±3%, but in another, after careful verification of the procedures and attention to detail, it may be entirely practicable to achieve precision of ±0.1% (absolute) in the analysis.

6.4 Spatial resolution

6.4.1 Introduction

Before we proceed to discuss spatial resolution in thin foil analysis, it will be as well that we understand exactly what we mean. In optical imaging, and indeed also electron optical instruments, the wave-nature of the radiation (be it photons or electrons) leads to the fundamental limit on the size of objects, or the distance between objects, that can be resolved. In elementary textbook treatments, it is always assumed that enough signal (photons, electrons, etc.) will be detected that signal-to-noise issues will be insignificant. In fact, this is not always so in the case of electron optical imaging. When imaging radiation sensitive materials, only so many electrons can bombard the sample before the essential details of the structure are masked or altered. Thus the number of electrons that can be used for creating the image may be severely limited; this places practical limits on the signal-to-noise ratio in the image, which in turn limits the ultimate spatial resolution. While this point is absolutely clear in texts devoted to the subject of radiation sensitive materials, most general discussions of image resolution in the electron microscope make no mention of it.

In X-ray analysis, we have already seen that the number of X-rays that can be detected places statistical limits on the analytical precision. The volume of sample generating the X-rays (which may be considered the 'spatial resolution') is clearly the volume which interacts with the beam; essentially, a cone extending through the sample with an initial diameter equal to the beam diameter, and increasing because of beam broadening as the electrons propagate through the specimen thickness. It transpires that when the beam diameter is brought to the optical limit, there is still enough information in the transmitted or scattered electrons to generate an electron image of the sample – to the extent that single atoms (of heavy metals) on a thin carbon film may be imaged – but the number of X-rays generated may be too small to provide a useful analysis. It will be necessary to compromise the dimensions of the interaction volume in order to get more analytical information.

Different analyses will require different X-ray counts, and hence different resolution compromises. Imagine a catalyst in the form of fine metallic particles supported on a substrate, which, for this discussion, we will ignore. Suppose the catalyst is made of equal amounts of two metallic components, let us say A and B, and the experimental requirement is to determine whether each particle is made up only of either A or B, or whether the two elements are present together in each particle, all of which can be assumed to have the same composition. Only a few counts will be required to achieve this goal. When we analyse a particle, the three possibilities are that we see X-rays only from A, only from B, or equal numbers from A and B. How many are needed to tell the difference? Suppose we have observed 10 counts from A, and none from B. (For the purposes of our example, we will overlook, for now, the question of whether 10 counts can be seen statistically above the background.) Let us compute how often we would be in error if we concluded that the particle contained only A. While 10 counts is really too small a number for Gaussian statistics to apply, we will stretch the approximation. The standard deviation is about 3 counts. Hence, if the sample were an equal mixture of A and B, we would expect to have seen 10 counts from B, which is three times the standard deviation from the observed number of zero. Statistically we expect a measurement to be within three standard deviations 99.5% of the time. If we repeated the measurement on 10 different particles, and each time measured only 10 counts of either A or B, and never saw both in a single particle, we would be justified in concluding that the particles were not alloyed, but consisted of pure metal. Thus a count rate of 1 count s^{-1} (leading to an acquisition time of 10 s for each spectrum) will satisfy our experimental need. Suppose now that the sample is prepared in a new way that results in the particles being alloyed, but with a varying composition. It is necessary to determine whether there is a systematic variation of the composition, at the 1% level, with size. It follows from the argument of Section 4.6 (though we do not derive it there) that to achieve this goal will require that 20 000 counts be acquired from each element in each particle – or a total count, not including the background, of 40 000. A far cry from the 10 counts required for the first analysis. As we shall see, if the particles are too small, this will not be achievable.

Special consideration must be given to the detection of segregation at interfaces – an important application of thin-foil microanalysis. However, before thinking about that, let us discuss the smallest volume of a sample from which we can obtain the required analytical data.

6.4.2 *Spatial resolution in thin foils*

From Equation 6.2 we know that the count rate is a function of the electron probe current and the sample thickness. All the other parameters of Equation 6.2 are either fundamental constants, or predetermined by the particular experiment. Thus the requirement of a minimum count rate for an experiment predetermines the minimum product of current and sample thickness. Since the beam will broaden as it passes through the sample, we need to minimize the thickness; however, as we might suppose that a corresponding increase of the probe current will entail an increase in the probe size, reducing the thickness too far will cause the resolution to be limited by the probe size. The best resolution, in terms of the minimum analysed volume, will therefore lie at some intermediate thickness and probe size.

It can indeed be shown that, in an optimized electron probe, the current i_p is given by an equation of the form:

$$i_p = \frac{\pi^2 \, d^{\frac{8}{3}} B}{(4C_s)^{\frac{2}{3}}}$$

(6.7)

where d is the probe diameter, C_s is the spherical aberration coefficient of the probe-forming lens and B is the brightness of the electron source. We should note that the derivation of this equation is not exact, and in other sources it can be found with slightly different constants, but the functional form is the same. The brightness of the electron source is a fundamental property, which is related to the total energy emitted per unit area of the emitter. The gun brightness cannot be increased without limit; different electron sources have different practicable brightnesses. Although brightness can be varied within some limits by compromises in the design, the three basic types of electron gun, that is, thermionic tungsten hairpins, thermionic LaB_6, and field emission, have approximate brightnesses respectively of 5, 200 and 10^4 V_o.A cm^{-2} Sr^{-1}, where V_o is the electron accelerating voltage. A steradian (Sr) is the unit of measurement of solid angle – the angle subtended at the centre of a sphere of unit radius by a unit area on the surface of the sphere.

We can see from Equation 6.7 that the maximum current in a given small probe can be obtained from a field-emission source, and microscopes fitted with such sources are inherently capable of the best spatial resolution in X-ray microanalysis. We may note though, that the maximum obtainable current from a field emitter is limited, by other factors, to a lower value than that from a LaB_6 source. Hence in applications requiring very high currents at larger probe sizes (when approximations used in the derivation of Equation 6.7 do not apply) the field-emission gun may actually give inferior performance. Thus, even if its high cost was not a factor, the field-emission gun would not always be the electron source of choice for a TEM.

The broadening of a medium-energy electron beam as it propagates through a sample has been the subject of both thought and practical experiment. The various available theories give generally similar results, and the experimental data do not have enough precision to distinguish between them. Thus most workers use what is termed the 'single-scattering' model, which states that the average diameter of an electron probe is given by:

$$b = 6.25 \cdot 10^5 \frac{Z}{E_o} \left(\frac{\rho}{A}\right)^{1/2} t^{3/2} \tag{6.8}$$

where Z is the atomic weight of the sample (mean atomic weight in the case of a compound), the other symbols have the meanings defined earlier in this chapter, and the beam broadening is given in centimetres. Several points should be made about this expression. Firstly, despite the appearance arising from illustrations accompanying the explanations in many texts, the expression gives an average diameter of the probe through the foil, not the diameter at the exit face. Secondly, 'average diameter' is defined as the diameter of a cylinder through the foil within which 90% of the X-rays are generated. Thirdly, this 'average diameter' may or may not give a realistic approximation of the signal obtained from an actual sample, depending on the geometry.

Let us make the approximation that the optimum spatial resolution is obtained when the beam broadening is equal to the initial probe diameter. Since the beam broadening depends on sample thickness, and the probe current depends on the beam diameter, this assumption relates the sample thickness and the probe current. Equation 6.2 therefore becomes a function of a single variable, which, if the values of the various quantities involved are taken from sources in the literature, can be solved for any required X-ray count rate. *Table 6.1* presents results published by Garratt-Reed for the case of analysis of Fe foils at different voltages and for different electron sources, and at different count rates. The advantages of the field-emission gun and of increasing the beam voltage are obvious.

Table 6.1. Optimum values, computed as described in the text, of electron probe diameter and sample thickness for an acquisition count rate of 2000 counts s^{-1}, from an Fe thin foil, to achieve best spatial resolution for microanalysis in a microscope with the indicated electron source (Garratt-Reed, 1986)

Electron energy (keV)	Thermionic tungsten		Cold field-emitter	
	Diameter (nm)	Thickness (nm)	Diameter (nm)	Thickness (nm)
100	14	88	1.8	22
300	9.5	138	1.2	35
500	7.7	168	1.0	42

Let us step back and consider what this result tells us. What we have actually computed is the minimum distance between point analyses for essentially independent results in a foil of appropriate thickness. This would be applicable to measuring, for example, a composition gradient in a sample. For example, *Figure 6.8* shows pearlite, which is a steel microstructure consisting of plates of cementite, a carbide phase, in a matrix of ferrite, which is relatively pure Fe. In the area of the illustration, the plates are perpendicular to the foil, which was prepared by ion-milling and is of relatively uniform thickness. The alloy contained about 2% Cr,

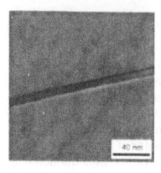

Figure 6.8. Micrograph of a cementite plate in pearlite, obtained at 100 kV (this is the area from which the plot of *Figure 6.13* was obtained).

which partitions during the growth of the pearlite to the cementite, although it is soluble in the ferrite. If held for a long time at high temperature, the Cr will diffuse to an equilibrium distribution with a high concentration in the cementite, and a low concentration in the ferrite. This sample, though, was quenched during the transformation, so no appreciable bulk diffusion of the Cr has taken place. We can thus measure the redistribution of the Cr during the growth of the pearlite.

Figure 6.9 shows a plot of the result of an analysis in a field-emission microscope at 250 keV electron energy, with a detector with a solid angle of 0.3 Sr. The data points have error bars representing a 2σ statistical uncertainty derived from the count rate. The solid line represents a plausible model of the actual Cr distribution, convoluted with a Gaussian of full-width at half-maximum of 1.2 nm. Except for small tails about 2 nm either side of the cementite, the agreement is seen to be excellent. The tails are believed to be due to spherical aberration – a problem we will address later. The count rate in this analysis was under 1000 counts s^{-1}, rather less than the high count-rate assumed in the derivation of *Table 6.1*, and the thickness of the sample is unknown; in any case because of the approximations, too much weight should not be placed on the fact that the resolution of *Figure 6.9* appears to exceed the prediction of *Table 6.1*. Nevertheless, it is apparent that *Table 6.1* does provide a realistic estimate of the resolution achievable in the analysis of foils.

6.4.3 Analysis of particles

Analysis of particles is a different problem. First we will consider the analysis of fine particles distributed on a thin support (such as a carbon film), which has negligible contrast in the image and negligible X-ray production. Since it must be possible to image the particle (in order to find it, to place the probe on it) the probe cannot be significantly larger than the particle. Assuming that there is enough contrast between the particle and the background, the electron probe diameter can be equal to the particle size; this will result in the maximum practicable count rate from the particle. Beam broadening will be negligible compared with the probe diameter. In this case, a different relationship is established between the

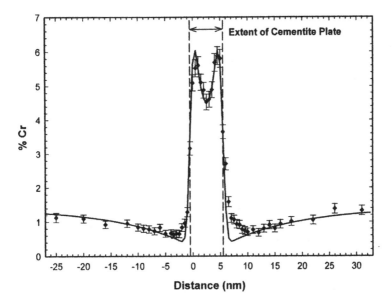

Figure 6.9. Plot of Cr composition against distance across a cementite plate in a Cr-containing pearlite at a beam voltage of 250 kV. The solid line represents a plausible model of the diffusion of the Cr, with realistic constraints, adjusted to fit the data, and convoluted with a Gaussian of FWHM of 1.2 nm.

probe diameter and the sample thickness (taken to be the particle diameter). Again, if desired, Equation 6.2 can be solved to obtain the optimum conditions.

In interpreting Table 6.1, it must be remembered that one assumption made during the derivation was that the electron probe was 'optimized'. This means that the convergence angle and demagnification have been appropriately adjusted for the required probe current. In fact, in many cases this will not be done. When analysing larger particles, the analyst will tend to leave the probe conditions fixed. The result is that most analyses of larger particles are 'sub-optimal' – at least in terms of this derivation of the theoretical count rates. Of course, in a practical situation, the contribution from the support will not usually be negligible, and may in some cases give significant interference in the analysis.

Analysis of particles in a thin foil presents a completely different set of challenges. Some possibilities are illustrated in *Figure 6.10*. If the particles all have different compositions, then the problem of performing quantitative analysis is essentially intractable. In the case of particles extending through the foil, of course (*Figure 6.10a*), the situation is just like the analysis of small regions of a thin foil, discussed in Section 6.4.2 above, provided that the analyst is certain that the particles do, in fact, extend through the foil. If there is some element present in the matrix which is not in the particle, then this is easy to determine – if the element is not present in the observed X-ray spectrum from the particle, then there is no overlap with the matrix and the analysis is from the particle. Otherwise, it will be necessary to use statistical methods. For example, if the composition of the matrix is X, and that of the particles (all of which are the same) is Y, then an analysis of particles will give a linear combination of X and Y – say, $AX + (1 - A)Y$. If a large number of analyses are obtained from different particles, the compositions will be found to extend from X towards Y. Assuming that some of the particles do, in fact, extend through the foil, a number of measurements will be found, all the same, taken from larger particles or in thinner parts of the foil, at the extreme of the composition range remote from the composition of the matrix. This extreme composition can be assumed to be that of the particles.

If no particles extend through the foil (*Figure 6.10b*), then quantitative analysis becomes far more difficult. Of course, if there is an element present in the matrix which is not present in the precipitate, then a spectrum obtained from the matrix can be normalized to this element in the spectrum from the precipitate, and then subtracted; the remaining spectrum is assumed to originate from the particle. Because of the statistical uncertainty introduced by the subtraction, the precision of the result may be poor, especially if the particle is small or if the element used for the normalization is not a major constituent of the matrix. The result is also dependent on there being no self-absorption of the X-rays in the sample.

Quantitative analysis in other cases (including the case of *Figure 6.10c*) is essentially impossible. The experimenter is probably best advised to find a way to separate the particles from the matrix. For example, in many metals, it is possible to make 'extraction replicas' which is a three-stage process; first, a polished surface of the sample is etched lightly so that the precipitates are left standing above the matrix. Secondly, a thin film of a suitable material – frequently, carbon – is deposited by evaporation or sputtering. Finally another etching step releases the precipitates completely from the matrix, so that they, embedded in the film, can be floated on the surface of a water bath and picked up on a fine support mesh. The resulting sample can then be placed in the microscope, and the problem becomes one of analysing particles on a thin substrate. It is

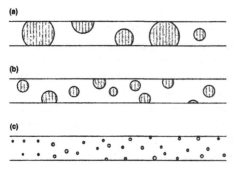

Figure 6.10. Sketch of different possibilities of particles embedded in thin foils. If the particles are of the same order as (or larger than) the foil thickness (a), then analysis can be relatively straightforward; if the particles are a moderate fraction of the sample thickness in size (b), then analysis may be possible, depending on the circumstances, while if the particles are very small (c), the analysis is essentially intractable, and other methods (such as preparing extraction replicas) should be considered.

necessary to consider the effect of the etch on the particles, any contamination introduced by a failure to remove the etching products completely from the film, and so on, but in many cases the needed data may be obtained from samples made in this way.

6.4.4 Analysis of interfaces

Segregation at interfaces in materials is very often of major interest. By 'interface' here we mean any planar structure such as a grain boundary or inter-phase interface. We must be clear, before continuing, that in this section we will be describing measurement of extremely narrow distributions at, or within a couple of atomic layers of, the actual boundary. In these cases, we cannot hope to resolve the actual solute distribution as a function of distance from the boundary (in fact, at this scale, because of the atomic structure of the solid, the interface itself may be considered to have a significant thickness). What we hope to obtain is a measurement of the total amount of segregation per unit area of the interface – the 'Gibbsian excess' solute. Composition gradients, such as diffusion profiles, extending from an interface into the material should be thought of as examples of high-resolution analysis of foils, discussed in Section 6.4.2.

Interface analysis is always attempted in the TEM by aligning the interface so that it is parallel with the electron beam. This is usually achieved by selecting an appropriate interface for analysis rather than by tilting the specimen (though a few degrees of adjustment may be applied to perfect the alignment). *Figure 6.11* shows the arrangement. A way to tell whether there is or is not segregation at the interface is simply to position the beam as shown in the illustration, and compare the resultant spectrum with a similar measurement taken from the matrix. Of course, if this is a phase interface, then it may be necessary to average spectra from the two phases, if they have different compositions. The presence of segregation is indicated, of course, by a difference between the spectra. It has been shown that this method is the most sensitive way to indicate the presence of segregation. The measured spectrum is not, of course, an analysis of the interface. The incident electron probe is probably larger than the 'width' of the interface, and beam broadening in the sample will contribute further

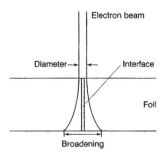

Figure 6.11. Sketch of the arrangement for detecting interface segregation.

matrix signal to the measurement. Hence it is difficult to relate the measured spectrum to an actual boundary segregation, although in cases of quite large changes in interface segregation it has proved possible to obtain useful relative measurements by this simple technique. Some efforts have been made to derive a quantitative measurement of interface segregation from these results, but they always depend on a knowledge of the sample thickness – which, as we have already noted, is very difficult to ascertain.

Two methods have been developed relatively recently to obtain quantitative measurements of the Gibbsian excess at narrow interfaces. One of these depends on X-ray mapping techniques; we will defer discussion of this method to Chapter 7, where we describe mapping. The other method depends on scanning the beam across a region of the interface.

The principal problem with quantification of interface segregation is to know the current density in the region of the sample. The current density varies because of the current profile in the incident probe, and varies with depth because of beam broadening. Suppose, though, what happens if the beam is scanned uniformly over a region large compared with the beam diameter and the broadening, as is illustrated in *Figure 6.12*. Assuming that the scan drive is linear, then, averaged over a large number of frames, each point within the scanned area, except for those points close to the edge, will receive the same amount of electron current, and the current density, similarly averaged over time, will be constant through the depth of the foil. Further, the electrons scattering away from the scanned region at the edges of the scanned area will compensate for the regions just inside the border of the area, in which the electron density is reduced. Thus the X-ray spectrum obtained is exactly the same as would have been obtained in a 'perfect' experiment by scanning over the same region in the absence of a finite probe diameter or beam broadening. Thus we are able to obtain an analysis of a rectangular slab of dimensions x, y, z. For the sake of simplicity, we will assume for this example that the matrix is a pure element, and that the segregant exists only at the interface. Clearly if these assumptions do not hold, modifications must be made to the following argument. The number of atoms in the slab is $x.y.z.\rho.N_o/A_m$, where ρ is the sample density, N_o is Avogadro's number and A_m is the atomic weight of the matrix, and we have assumed that the number of segregant atoms is small. If an interface of area $x.z$ bisects the slab, as shown in *Figure 6.12*, then there will be some segregant atoms in the slab. The X-ray signal from the segregant will be detected during the analysis, and can be quantified, leading to a ratio R of segregant atoms to matrix atoms. Hence the number of segregant atoms is $R.x.y.z.\rho.N_o/A_m$. Since the area of the interface is $x.z$, the number of atoms per unit area is $R.y.\rho.N_o/A_m$. This is the required Gibbsian segregation, and may be immediately calculated because all the parameters of the expression are known.

Since the electron beam is deliberately spread out during this analysis, the signal detected from the interface is relatively small. Hence it is necessary to count for a long time – typically several hundred seconds – to

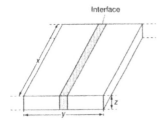

Figure 6.12. Sketch showing how scanning the electron probe over a region including the interface can lead to a quantitative measurement of the Gibbsian segregation.

obtain satisfactory counting statistics. One of the advantages of scanning the beam is that an image is obtained on the screen throughout the analysis, so drift of the image may be monitored and corrected.

The appropriate distance to scan the beam will vary with the sample thickness. Since the goal is to eliminate the need to know the sample thickness for each analysis, a suitable scan geometry for the maximum anticipated thickness must be chosen. Exactly how this is done is up to the user to decide. For example, in the authors' case, it has been shown that under specific analytical conditions, a particular count rate is obtained in the X-ray detector from an Fe foil sample about 100 nm thick. The single-scattering model estimates the beam broadening in this thickness of Fe at 250 kV to be 7 nm. Remembering that the beam broadening is the diameter of the profile, we can see that if we keep the count rate below this value (for the predefined beam conditions – i.e. beam limiting aperture and condenser lens settings, emission current, etc., and for the same pulse processor time constant) then it is satisfactory to scan 8 nm either side of the interface, that is, over a total area 16×16 nm.

Deriving an approximate detection limit for this type of analysis is difficult, because by the nature of the experiment, the conditions are variable. However, if R is 0.001, and y is 20 nm, then the number of atoms on the boundary would be about 2×10^{13} cm^{-2}. For comparison, a close-packed layer in Fe contains about 2×10^{15} atoms cm^{-2}. Experiments have generally shown this rough calculation to be about right.

6.5 Microscope considerations

It is not the purpose of this book to describe the operation of the electron microscope. However, as has been pointed out several times in the last sections, it is important that the electron probe be 'optimized', and we will spend a few paragraphs discussing what this means.

There are three contributions to the width of an electron probe; diffraction, spherical aberration and geometrical (i.e. the demagnification of the physical source size onto the sample). The diffraction contribution goes as the inverse of the probe convergence angle; the spherical aberration limit goes as the third power of the angle. The smallest achievable size is set, approximately, when these two are equal. This is the resolution limit described in textbooks. The maximum current is obtained in this probe when the demagnification is set so that the geometrical probe size is also equal to the spherical aberration and diffraction contributions.

To obtain more current in the probe it is necessary to increase the probe convergence angle, so the diffraction limit is not significant. However, as the spherical aberration goes as the cube of the convergence the probe size increases very rapidly with convergence. Thus it is very important to match the geometrical probe size with the spherical aberration to obtain an optimized probe. How this is done will vary from instrument to instrument. Some general principles can be given, though. The demagnification is controlled by the settings of the condenser lenses. The probe current and convergence angle are both determined by the probe-forming aperture – although at least one of these quantities will also be affected by the settings of the condenser lenses. Hence every adjustment of the probe current will require different aperture and condenser settings. The analyst must study the electron optics of the particular instrument to determine what these settings are. For the purposes of probe formation, there is only one appropriate setting of the lenses for each available probe-limiting aperture. There is nothing to be gained (and potentially much to lose) by not operating with these optimum settings when performing X-ray analysis. Note that this statement does not apply necessarily to other applications of the instrument in which other operating conditions may indeed be appropriate.

It is critically important that the probe-limiting aperture be accurately centred. *Figure 6.13* is an analysis of the same sample (not the same area) as was illustrated in *Figure 6.9*, but with an off-centre probe-limiting aperture. (To set the record completely straight, we must add that the results were not obtained in the same microscope, either, but that does not affect our conclusions.) The details of the profile in *Figure 6.13* are substantially hidden. This is because very small changes in the aperture position cause remarkably large changes in the probe profile, especially when operating the microscope at the maximum beam convergence. It should be mentioned that the aperture alignment for the measurement of *Figure 6.13* had been performed in accordance with the operator's instructions. Only after this measurement was made was it found that the instructions actually led to a subtle misalignment of the aperture. For the best results, it is essential that this type of subtlety be well characterized. Likewise the focus setting is critical. The larger the probe convergence, the more under focus the lens must be to be optimized. However, the larger the convergence, the more quickly the probe size increases with defocus. Focusing cannot, in general, be performed on the bright-field image, because it is not sensitive enough to the defocus. The annular dark-field image must be used. This is a problem for users of microscopes without annular dark-field capability. For the same reason, focus stability is absolutely critical for the best analysis.

If a compromise must be made, or if there is any possibility that the microscope parameters are not accurately known, the operator should

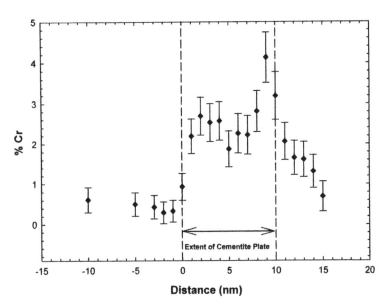

Figure 6.13. Plot of Cr concentration as a function of position across the cementite plate shown in *Figure 6.8.* The asymmetric form was subsequently shown to have been due to misalignment of the probe-limiting aperture. If the aperture had been properly aligned, a plot similar to *Figure 6.9* would have been expected.

always ensure that the probe convergence angle is kept below the target value. The sensitivity of the probe size to the adjustments arises because of the third power dependence of the spherical aberration on convergence angle. Reducing the convergence angle provides a margin for error, if such a margin is needed.

In concluding this chapter, we will say a few words about the difference between a TEM/STEM and a dedicated STEM. A TEM/STEM is an instrument in which either a conventional image of the sample may be formed, or a fine electron probe may be formed and scanned on the sample. The dedicated STEM, in contrast, has only a scanning mode of operation. Until recently, at least, the dedicated STEM has provided the best analytical performance from thin samples. This, though, is not because of any fundamental inability of the TEM/STEM to offer the same performance. Rather, it is because of the pressure on manufacturers to provide ultra-high resolution imaging performance in a TEM/STEM. This requirement leads to compromises in other areas, amongst which are probe-forming and analytical capability. A different set of compromises would lead instead to a superior probe-forming analytical instrument, with good, but not outstanding, TEM imaging capability. No manufacturer has yet been induced to build such an instrument!

7 X-ray mapping

7.1 Introduction

An X-ray map produced from an electron microscope is nothing more than an image of the sample formed from a selected (and possibly processed) part of the X-ray spectrum. There are several reasons why this is very valuable. A common application is as a qualitative 'screening' to identify relatively gross variations in the composition in different parts of a sample, which may then be subjected to more detailed examination. In a large image it can often be difficult to find features of interest; if there is a compositional variation that can be mapped, then the map can show these. Sometimes the map can show an unexpected feature that would not have been found otherwise. In other cases the map provides access to information that would otherwise be hard to determine. A very significant attribute is that the map presents the analytical data in a powerful, easy to interpret way that makes a strong impact on a scientific audience. The saying 'a picture is worth a thousand words' applies here. The analyst not only has to determine the composition of the sample, but that information must be transmitted to an audience. Even if all the quantitative data have been acquired by other means, the map can still present this in a simple way, making the time spent recording it worthwhile. Other important applications, which we shall discuss during the course of this chapter, have also been developed.

7.2 Hardware implementation

All modern probe-forming microscopes (SEMs and STEMs) have the ability to control the probe position by the application of external voltages driving the scan circuitry. The most usual implementation of X-ray mapping uses digital-to-analogue converters in the X-ray analyser computer to generate the scan voltages. This computer is then used for all the acquisition tasks. In some cases, the X-ray analysis program may in fact be running on the same computer as the microscope control, and there may be more or less integration between the various components of the software. However, the essential functions will remain the same. As very few users implement their own interfacing of the computer to the microscope, and the hardware details are unimportant for the application of mapping, we will not discuss them further.

Some older microscopes may not have provision for accepting an external scan drive. The analyst then has two options (if one discounts replacing the microscope!). Either an electronic specialist can be enlisted to conduct surgery on the microscope circuitry to provide external drive capability (in many cases entirely practical for an experienced engineer, but fraught with pitfalls for the inexperienced), or an external acquisition system capable of making use of the microscope's own scan generator can be acquired. This latter course works well for digital image acquisition, but has disadvantages (principally, significant lack of operational flexibility) for mapping.

In the most typical case, the user will define one or more regions of interest (or 'windows') in the X-ray spectrum – usually corresponding to the energies of the X-rays from elements of interest (in much the same way as windows can be defined, as described in Chapter 4, to determine the intensity of the X-ray peaks). The computer will then scan the electron probe over the sample area, dwelling for some pre-defined time at each pixel, during which an X-ray spectrum is acquired. At the end of the pre-selected dwell time, the numbers of X-rays detected in each window (and, usually, in order to obtain an electron image simultaneously, the detected electron intensity), are saved to memory, before the probe moves to the next pixel and the process is repeated. The entire dataset is eventually written to disk. Modern software typically provides a number of options for presenting or processing the data, and it is also most convenient if an option is available for exporting the images in a standard form (such as TIFF). A typical X-ray map, together with a secondary electron image is shown in *Figure 7.1* – in this case, the distribution of Pb and Sn in a sample of Pb–Sn solder. The maps of Pb and Sn are shown, and it can readily be seen that there are two phases, of which the Pb-rich phase appears to be islands in a Sn-rich matrix.

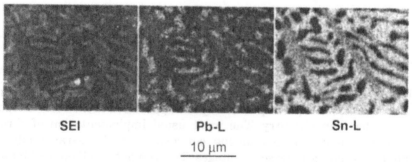

| SEI | Pb-L | Sn-L |

10 μm

Figure 7.1. Secondary electron image (left), with X-ray maps of Pb-L (centre) and Sn-L (right) obtained from a sample of solder in an SEM at 30 kV. The Pb-rich regions appear to be islands in a Sn-rich matrix.

We may note that as we describe the process here, we assume that the area of the image is scanned once, dwelling for the desired time at each pixel. This is not necessarily the case. It is equally possible to scan the area multiple times, dwelling at each pixel for only a fraction of the total time each scan, and summing the results in the computer. The disadvantage of using multiple scans arises mainly in the STEM when mapping at extremely high magnification, when the image might drift from scan to scan, causing the features to be smeared in the maps. The drift would still distort the image during a single scan, but the features would be sharp (assuming the microscope was focused). The advantage of the multiple scan technique is that the operator can see if anything interesting is becoming visible in the images and can terminate the scan or choose to continue as appropriate, rather than having to just wait for the whole acquisition to finish.

7.3 Statistical considerations

The numbers of counts recorded in each pixel are typically not large. This is a consequence of the very large number of pixels in even a modest image, and in turn determines the information that is accessible by mapping. For example, a 128 × 128 image contains 16 384 pixels. If the dwell time (the acquisition time) for each pixel was 100 ms, then, allowing for detector dead time and system overhead, it will take about half an hour to acquire a map with this resolution. Consider that a 'moderate' count rate for spectrum acquisition in an SEM would be about 4000 counts s^{-1}. Hence 400 counts will be recorded in 100 ms, of which about half, or about 200, as we have already seen, will be in the major peak of the spectrum (assuming the specimen contains a single dominant element and some trace elements). Since we are recording unprocessed X-ray counts, we will record bremsstrahlung as well as characteristic X-rays. Hence we must take account of the background in interpreting the image. The background in the peak window will be typically about 6% of counts in the major peak, or about 12 counts. A trace element present at the level of 1% will add about 2 counts to this background. While in a spectrum with good signal to noise ratio this signal would be easily detectable, it may not be in a map. A further problem introduced by the background is that it varies in intensity with the sample composition (and, in the case of mapping in the TEM, with the sample thickness). When attempting to map an element present at low levels in a sample, it is useful to define a window in the spectrum selected to sample the background only. If the details in the elemental map and the background map are (within the limits set by the available counts) the same, then the background variation is dominating the elemental map, and no conclusions about the distribution of that element can be drawn.

In the TEM the peak to background ratio of the X-ray peaks is larger than in the SEM, so it might be expected that mapping in the TEM would be sensitive to smaller concentrations of trace elements. If maps are acquired at equal X-ray count rates, this expectation is indeed met. However, even 4000 counts s^{-1} is a higher count rate than is employed for most quantitative analysis in the TEM (as was discussed in Chapter 6). To achieve this rate it will normally be necessary to use thicker areas of the sample and/or larger electron probe sizes. Either alternative involves re-adjustment of the microscope, which might be undesirable because of other constraints of the investigation.

While X-ray mapping is not especially useful for illustrating distributions of trace elements, it is, on the other hand, excellent at illustrating small regions where the trace elements are concentrated. For example, *Figure 7.2* shows a map of a steel sample, containing about 1 wt% Mo. The pixel acquisition time was far too short to show the bulk Mo content; however, in the Mo map, we see small regions with great enrichment of Mo. These are in fact carbides. In the electron image (also shown in *Figure 7.2*), some of these are clearly visible, but others would probably be missed in the dense array of dislocations.

Because of the small number of counts recorded in each pixel, the acquisition of an X-ray map is almost always a compromise between spatial resolution, sensitivity, time, and, perhaps, sample degradation. In the SEM, it is helpful to remember that the spatial resolution of the analysis is rarely much better than 1 μm; thus there is little point in acquiring a map with pixels spaced, say 10 nm apart. Likewise, there is no point in operating the instrument in a high-resolution imaging mode (implying a small current) because the use of a larger probe, with more current, will not degrade the practical spatial resolution of the map at all. In fact, in virtually all analytical situations when the sample is stable (i.e. not suffering from damage caused by the beam), the best maps will be obtained when the beam current is

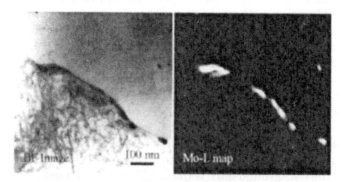

Figure 7.2. Bright-field image (left) and Mo-L X-ray map obtained from a low-alloy steel in a STEM at 250 kV. Several Mo-rich precipitates are apparent, both on the interface and in the matrix. Comparison between the bright-field image and the map shows that some of the precipitates, which are obvious in the map, are not clearly visible in the electron image.

increased so that the detector is operating at about 50% dead time – which is about the maximum rate of collection of X-ray data in real time. Also, the pulse processing time should normally be set as short as possible, again to maximize the number of counts acquired – the loss in spectral resolution is more than compensated for by the increase in the signal.

7.3.1 Examples

We can illustrate these effects with a series of simulations, shown in *Figure 7.3*. In each case the image size is 128 × 128 pixels; the upper image of each pair shows a feature 64 × 64 pixels centred in the image, and the lower image shows four 8 × 8 pixel features centred in each quadrant of the main image. All the images have been adjusted so that the overall grey level is approximately the same (as would probably be done in practice).

In *Figure 7.3a* we show a simulation of the situation described in the first paragraph of section 7.3 above, in which a feature present at the 1% level is superimposed on the background. The larger feature is visible, though not outstandingly so; the four smaller features, though, would most likely be missed in examining the image without the foreknowledge of their presence. *Figure 7.3b* shows an image modelled with 0.5 counts (on average) in the bremsstrahlung, and an extra 0.5 counts in the feature. This might represent a STEM map of a moderately thin foil, with a feature present at the 1% level. Again, the larger feature is clear, but the smaller features would probably be missed. An obvious additional lesson to be learned from this simulation is that a feature can be seen even if the counts in each individual pixel are not significant. In the background there are many pixels with two or more counts recorded, and in the feature there are many pixels with no counts. It is only by averaging the information (in this case, by the use of the eye and the brain's averaging powers) that the presence of the feature is seen. *Figure 7.3c* shows the same simulated

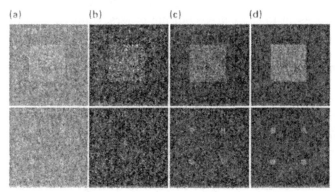

Figure 7.3. Simulation (using a random-number generator) of noisy X-ray maps. The upper row shows a single large feature, while the lower row shows four smaller features, one in each quadrant. The large feature is clearly more obvious. The number of counts and the signal-to-noise ratio are different for each pair of simulations. See the text for more details.

situation, but with three times more counts recorded. The features are more visible, but only marginally so. It is only when recording 10 times more counts (*Figure 7.3d*) that a major improvement in the image quality is perceived.

In contrast, a major composition variation, such as the molybdenum carbides discussed above, is easily observed. In *Figure 7.4* is a simulation of small features, 2 × 2 pixels, in which the X-ray counts are significantly (in the statistical sense) above the background. It can be seen that they stand out obviously.

Figure 7.4. Similar to the lower row of *Figure 7.3*, but with higher signal-to-noise. See the text for details.

7.3.2 *Spectral overlaps*

Spectral overlaps present a difficult problem in X-ray mapping. All spectral deconvolution techniques, as discussed in Chapter 4, require good counting statistics for successful application; in mapping applications, such statistics are rarely, if ever available. Mapping another line for one of the elements and subtracting is unlikely to be successful because, even if the count rates for the X-rays of the element in the two windows could be made equal on average, again the statistics would dominate the final image (in statistical terms, subtraction has exactly the same effect on the uncertainty as addition, only now the imprecision is in the small difference between the two numbers, rather than in the larger sum of them). The best that can be done is to present a subjective view, showing that one element is present in some areas but not others, while the second appears everywhere. More careful analysis must be performed to clarify the chemistry. *Figure 7.5*, which shows maps from an integrated circuit (in which the silicon and tungsten result in a peak overlap) illustrates the point.

7.4 Other applications

X-ray mapping is capable of revealing quite subtle features of a sample, mainly because of the ability of the eye to average information, as we mentioned earlier. Consider a particle with a coating. A simple point analysis of the particle will average the coating and the bulk. However, if we consider the analysis at the centre and at the edge of the particle, the

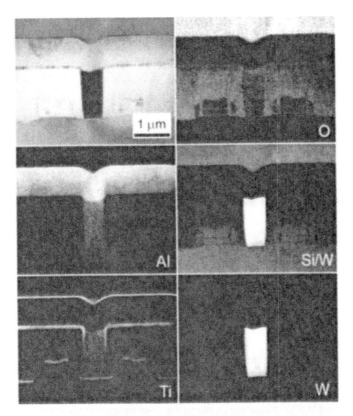

Figure 7.5. Bright-field image and elemental maps as indicated from an integrated circuit observed in a STEM at 250 kV. W has a characteristic line that overlaps the Si K line. Hence the bright feature in the centre of the Si/W map, which corresponds to the bright region of the W map, cannot be assumed to contain Si/W (in fact, separate spectral analysis indicates that it does not). Other regions of the Si/W map that are moderately bright, where the W map is dark, do correspond to Si-containing regions of the sample.

results will be clearly different, because at the centre the core of the particle has maximum thickness, while the coating is sampled with the minimum projected thickness. Close to the edge the reverse is true. This is shown in *Figure 7.6*, together with a simulation of an X-ray map (both of the core and the coating) from such a particle. In a colour overlay, not practicable to reproduce in this book, the difference is particularly striking. Nevertheless, the different form of the maps is quite obvious. *Figure 7.7* shows an example, of Mg particles with an oxide layer on the surface. While this information could also be obtained by conducting, for example, a line-scan, that requires a foreknowledge of what features might be present in the sample, while the map shows whatever is there, provided only that the correct elements have been chosen for the acquisition.

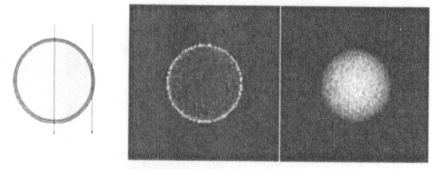

Figure 7.6. Drawing of analysis of a coated sphere (left), with simulations of X-ray maps of the coating material (centre) and the core (right), showing very obvious differences in appearance.

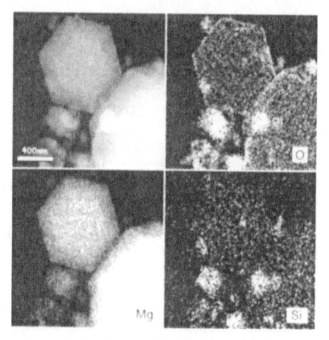

Figure 7.7. Annular dark-field image (upper left), with O (upper right), Mg (lower left) and Si (lower right) maps of Mg metal particles, imaged in a STEM at 250 kV. The distribution of O on the Mg particles is seen to correspond (qualitatively) with the simulation of *Figure 7.6*, and it is therefore deduced that the O is simply present in a thin surface oxide. The Si, evidently present in oxide particles, is an unwanted contaminant (illustration courtesy of A. Diaz and A. Sarofim, MIT).

7.4.1 Spectral imaging

Even this last condition can be relaxed in a form of mapping known as 'spectral imaging'. In this technique, the entire X-ray spectrum from the sample is stored for each pixel. If we had been writing this monograph a few years ago, we might have described the memory, and especially the hard disk space, required for such an acquisition as 'prodigious', or some similar adjective, for a 128 × 128 pixel map, storing a 1024-point X-ray spectrum with a maximum count of 255 (1 byte) at each channel, requires 16 megabytes of storage. A 256 × 256 pixel map, storing two bytes of X-ray data at each channel, needs 128 megabytes of disk space. The advantage, though, is that the data can be re-visited if, for example, it appears that an extra element should be added to the map. If several hours have been invested in the acquisition, this capability can be a major advantage. Only very recently (at the time of writing) have commercial systems with spectral mapping capability become available.

7.4.2 *Quantitative X-ray mapping*

Most X-ray mapping applications are purely qualitative – the position of any compositional variations is revealed, but only in the roughest sense is any indication given as to the quantitative analysis at any point, especially as it is usual to adjust the contrast of each map individually to give good visibility of the details. However, this need not be the case, there being a number of ways that mapping can be employed to give quantitative results.

One way to use mapping as a quantitative tool is to acquire enough counts at each pixel that a quantitative analysis may be performed; the result of the analysis is then stored at the pixel position in the map. While the result at any individual pixel is necessarily uncertain (because of the limited dwell time at that pixel, of course), by averaging over appropriate areas, the precision can be improved. For example, it is possible to take a 10 × 10 pixel region within a grain, and obtain an analysis that is comparable with that obtained by analysing the grain for 100 times the pixel dwell time. Likewise, if a grain boundary or other interface shows segregation, then averaging the composition along lines parallel to the interface can give a high-resolution line-scan across the interface. This in turn can lead to a determination of the quantitative amount of segregation (in terms of atoms of segregant per unit area of interface). *Figure 7.8*, reproduced by courtesy of Masashi Watanabi and David B. Williams, shows a quantitative map of yttrium segregation at grain boundaries in zirconia. Carpenter *et al.* have derived grain boundary segregation measurements from similar maps acquired from Al–Cu samples by averaging the quantitative analysis over some distance along interfaces to generate average composition profiles.

We note that this last result could equally have been obtained by spectral imaging. Composition values obtained along lines parallel with the interface could be integrated, leading to compound profiles of high precision, from which could then be derived the same compositional line-scan across the interface. We are assuming, of course, that there is no significant compositional variation along the interface when performing this averaging.

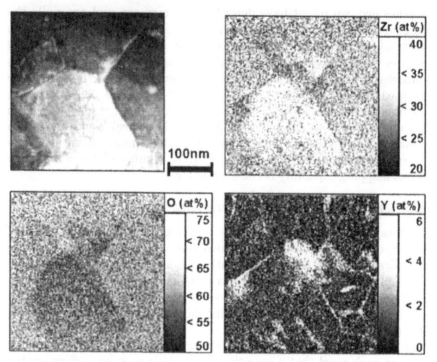

Figure 7.8. Quantitative X-ray map, obtained in a STEM at 300 kV, of Y in zirconia, showing the Y segregation at the grain boundaries. Further processing of such maps can lead to a quantitative estimate of the Gibbsian segregation at the interface (illustration courtesy of M. Watanabe and D. B. Williams, Lehigh University).

Another way of using X-ray mapping in a quantitative way relies on a totally different idea. The electron microscope is often employed as a tool for making quantitative measurements of different phases in a sample. Unfortunately, though, it can sometimes be quite difficult to determine from the electron image which part of the sample is which phase. By using X-ray mapping, compositional variations between the phases can lead to identification of the regions. Even if the data are relatively noisy, image analysis procedures are readily available to average the noise and to compute the area of the image occupied by each phase. *Figure 7.9* shows an example, from the work of Pint *et al.*, in which very fine zirconium oxide particles are growing on the surface of an alumina film. A STEM sample has been prepared by thinning from the back of the alumina (i.e. the side away from the zirconia particles). It was desired to use digital image processing to determine the number and size of the zirconia particles, and the fraction of the surface covered by them. Given the thickness variation of the alumina film and the contrast variation from grain to grain, it was not easily possible to segment the electron image to determine where the zirconia particles were, but the zirconium X-ray map showed them clearly, allowing the size and number to be tracked according to the experimental conditions.

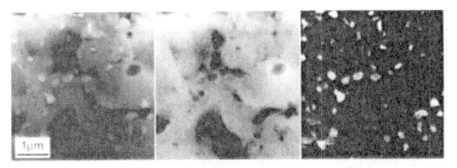

Figure 7.9. Annular dark-field image (left) with Al (centre) and Zr (right) X-ray maps, obtained in a STEM at 100 KV, of the oxide scale formed on a Zr-doped Ni–Al alloy. Most of the zirconia particles are visible in the electron image, but image analysis was unable to identify them reliably. In contrast, it was able to identify and measure the particles in the Zr map. Ratioing the area of the particles to the area of the alumina (determined from the alumina map) gave the fractional coverage of the surface, allowing for the fact that there were some holes in the sample within the field of view (from the work of B. A. Pint, A. J. Garratt-Reed and L. W. Hobbs, MIT).

7.5 Concluding comments

We have discussed the mechanics of X-ray mapping, pointing out that it is not, except in special cases, a quantitative technique. We have shown some examples of X-ray maps, and discussed some applications. In ending this chapter, we will refer back to the Pb–Sn solder sample used in *Figure 7.1*. In chapter 5 we discussed the spatial resolution of X-ray analysis in the SEM. We described how the electrons penetrate the surface of, and spread within, the sample, and generate X-rays from the entire region. We did not, though, show an illustration at that time, rather referring ahead to this section.

In *Figure 7.10* we show more X-ray maps acquired from the same area as *Figure 7.1*. In particular *Figure 7.10a* (the same as *Figure 7.1a*) is a map of the Pb L X-rays (about 10.55 keV) at a beam energy of 30 keV; *Figure 7.10b* shows the same area, but the Pb M X-rays (about 2.35 keV) mapped with a beam energy of 8 keV. *Figure 7.10c* shows Cu K X-rays (8.04 keV) and *Figure 7.10d* Cu L X-rays (0.93 keV), in the same conditions as *Figure 7.10a* and *7.10b*, respectively. Finally *Figure 7.10e* shows a secondary electron image in the same condition as *Figure 7.10a*, and *Figure 7.10f* a backscattered electron image in the same condition as *Figure 7.10b*. Comparison of *Figures 7.10a* and *7.10b* demonstrates immediately the improvement in spatial resolution obtained by reducing the electron beam voltage, as we described in chapter 5. By looking critically, it is possible to see that several of the Pb-rich regions that appear separate in *Figure 7.10b* are in fact joined together beneath the sample surface, because in *Figure 7.10a* there are indistinct and less intense Pb responses. Reference back to *Figure 7.1b* shows that Sn is present in these regions (it is not possible to

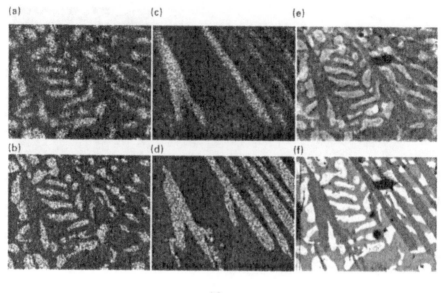

10 µm

Figure 7.10. The same sample and area as *Figure 7.1.* The upper row shows, from left to right, the Pb L map, the Cu K map, and the secondary electron image in the same conditions as *Figure 7.1* (i.e. 30 KV electron beam). The lower row shows, respectively, the Pb M map, the Cu L map, and the backscattered electron image, acquired at 8 KV beam energy. Not only is the spatial resolution clearly better in the lower row, with the lower beam energy and the lower energy X-ray lines, but, as described in the text, comparison of the two rows makes it clear that the Cu is present only in moderately thin sheets on the surface.

obtain a useful map of the Sn distribution at a beam energy of 8 keV because the Sn L X-ray lines are not excited sufficiently strongly). Likewise, the difference in the resolution is very obvious in the Cu maps, but these tell us more, too. While the intensity of the Cu signal is quite uniform in the low-energy map, some parts in the high-energy map are more intense than others, because the high-energy electrons are able to penetrate the Cu region (actually, undoubtedly a Cu–Sn alloy), and therefore generate fewer X-rays. Further, a careful inspection of the high-energy Pb map shows that in some cases the Pb-rich phase is visible underneath the Cu-rich regions. Hence we can deduce that the Cu-rich regions are thin layers on the surface of the sample.

This series of illustrations is an excellent example, therefore, of two of the principal attributes of the power of X-ray maps: the power to demonstrate in an easily-interpreted, visual way, some feature of the analysis (in this case, the improved spatial resolution of X-ray analysis at low electron energies), and the very large amount of information gathered which leads to interpretations that would not otherwise be readily apparent.

8 Energy-dispersive X-ray analysis compared with other techniques

8.1 Introduction

EDX analysis is not the only technique available for microanalysis of samples. In this chapter we will endeavour to make comparisons between EDX and other similar microanalysis techniques and in conclusion evaluate the strengths and shortcomings of EDX compared with other microanalysis methods. This list is not exhaustive and a more comprehensive listing of materials analysis techniques can be found in Brundle and Evans (1992).

Any particular analysis technique has its strengths, and in practice the question that should be asked is, 'What information do I require?' The answer usually narrows the possible techniques to only a few, and then it becomes a matter of convenience, sometimes cost and equipment availability.

8.2 Wavelength-dispersive X-ray analysis – electron probe microanalysis (EPMA)

Wavelength-dispersive spectroscopy (WDS) is the most directly comparable technique to EDX; both use electron-excited X-rays to allow characterization of a sample. The two techniques are often combined in EPMA (*Figure 8.1*) to form a highly quantitative microanalysis system, which takes advantage of the strengths of both methods. An EPMA system usually consists of the following:

- An electron probe forming system able to produce beam currents between pA and μA and beam diameters from nm to μm.
- One or several WDS and an EDX spectrometer.
- A high-vacuum system usually in the 10^{-6} Pa range.
- Computer system to acquire and analyse the data.

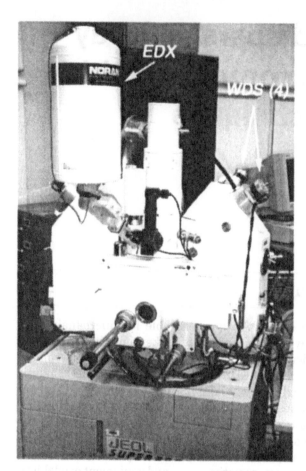

Figure 8.1. A typical electron microprobe, a JEOL JXA-8900 SUPERPROBE, showing the WDS spectrometers, of which there are four (two arrowed) and an EDX detector. The WDS spectrometers have motors on the top of them to drive the mechanical scans (illustration courtesy of Peter McSwiggen, Geology Department, University of Minnesota).

Of specific interest in this discussion is the operation and specifications of the WDS and its comparison to the EDX. WDS is based upon the Bragg diffraction of X-rays incident on an analysing crystal, which forms part of the WDS detector. The WDS focuses the X-rays from the sample onto the slit of a detector, using a curved crystal, which diffracts the X-rays according to the Bragg equations. The wavelength that is diffracted is adjusted by a mechanical movement of the crystal and detector. Hence only a single wavelength can be detected at any instant, the full spectrum being obtained by a slow scanning of the spectrometer. It is necessary to use a selection of different crystals, of different lattice-spacing, to get effective coverage of the entire X-ray wavelength range of interest for general-purpose analysis. Hence EPMAs typically have several (three or more) spectrometers, each fitted with a different crystal. Of course, for a specific application it may not be necessary to use three crystals, and an instrument dedicated to a single application may have only one or two spectrometers.

The major strengths and weaknesses of WDS compared to EDX can be summarized as follows and as illustrated in *Figure 8.2.*

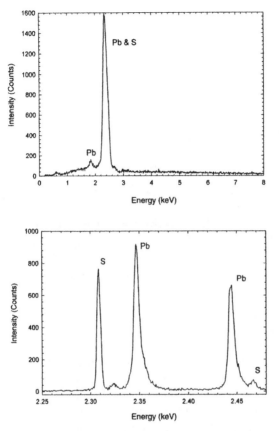

Figure 8.2. (Top) EDX spectrum of galena (PbS) showing the overlap of Pb and S peaks, (bottom) equivalent WDS spectrum showing the clear separation of the Pb and S peaks. Acquisition time for the EDX spectra was 20 s, whereas the WDS acquisition required 200 s (illustration courtesy of Peter McSwiggen, Geology Department, University of Minnesota).

8.2.1 Spectral resolution

In WDS, the FWHM of an X-ray peak is limited by crystal imperfections and the mechanical scanning available in the system to about 10 eV. In EDX, the resolution is limited by charge carrier statistics and analysis limits the resolution to about 130 eV, thus WDS wins by a factor of 10 in terms of spectral resolution.

8.2.2 Peak to background

Because peak to background is directly related to spectral resolution, the more sharply defined WDS peaks means that the peak to background is proportionally higher, the background being smaller for WDS since the peak is spread over a smaller energy range. The detection limit for WDS is typically 100 ppm, whereas for EDX it is approximately 100–200 ppm.

8.2.3 Spectral acquisition

The main advantage in EDX analyis is that it can measure any X-ray that reaches the detector, and can continually measure the entire X-ray spectrum; the WDS must be mechanically scanned over differing ranges (and angles) with several crystal changes. If an unknown element is present then the EDX in an EPMA system is used first to identify the elements present before the WDS is used. In this case the EDX is used to perform a rapid qualitative analysis.

8.2.4 Dead time and counting rate

For EDX the time constant is of the order of 10–50 μs and for WDS is 0.05–0.1 μs; hence, the WDS detector can count much faster. Since WDS makes use of diffraction to disperse the X-rays before entering the detector, the limiting count rate for WDS applies to a single characteristic X-ray, whereas for EDX it applies to the whole spectrum. This makes detecting trace elements a more difficult measurement with EDX than WDS.

8.2.5 Geometrical considerations

As WDS uses a wavelength spectrometer, the alignment of the instrument with respect to the sample and hence the source of the X-rays is of critical importance. Uniform X-ray transmission occurs within an ellipsoid of particular volume; the long axis has dimensions of the order of 100–1000 μm, while the short axis is only 10 μm. On a dedicated EPMA system, this is achieved by incorporating an optical microscope or scope camera to ensure the sample is positioned at the required alignment point. The advantage with EDX is that the geometrical considerations are not as stringent, since the EDX itself is a non-focusing device and sample placement is adjusted to usually achieve maximum X-ray intensity.

8.3 Electron energy-loss spectroscopy (EELS)

EELS measures energy lost after a highly energetic electron passes through a sample. As a result, the method can directly detect the energy used to create a characteristic X-ray: EELS is the primary interaction event detection method. EELS is an analytical technique used on the TEM, although there is a version that is used for reflection electron energy-loss measurements (REELS). EELS is an absorption spectroscopy, and the elemental information in the sample is derived from elemental edge profiles and arises from the excitation of discrete inner shell electrons above the Fermi level. EELS can give local elemental concentration of each atomic species, in the same way as EDX can. EELS can also supply information about chemical bonding, electronic structure and average nearest-neighbour distances (albeit with a great deal of effort!).

Quantification of concentrations for EELS are quoted to about 1–2 at%, whereas detection limits are down to ~10^{-21} g, depending on the elements involved. The biggest advantage when using EELS as compared to EDX is in performing spatially resolved analysis from sample areas in the order of 10 Å or less, dependent on the optics. A major advantage of using EELS is its ability to detect and measure light elements – all the way to H (at least in theory – in practice, measurements of H and Li can often be difficult). EELS does not suffer from the limitations of X-ray absorption of light elements as in EDX. The spectral resolution of EELS peaks and edges are in the order of tenths of an electron volt, whereas the spectral resolution of EDX systems is of the order of 130 eV. The greatest advantage in EDX analysis over EELS is that the entire spectrum can be acquired in one pass, whereas to acquire the complete elemental information the EELS spectrum usually requires several passes at differing energy offsets, depending on the requirements of the particular analysis.

EELS has a higher signal, but also has a higher background that has to be fitted and removed. EELS has a higher ultimate spatial resolution, but only when a very thin sample has been made. Perhaps the single most important disadvantage of EELS is that it is much more operator dependent, with fitting and deconvolution needed to extract even the most basic quantitative information. *Figure 8.3* compares an EELS spectrum

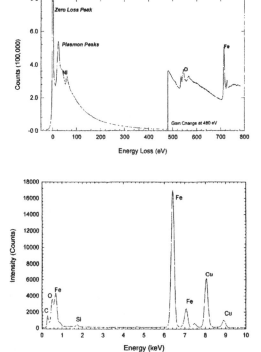

Figure 8.3. (Top) EELS spectrum obtained in a TEM/STEM at 200 KV from an iron oxide-based meteorite. Note the gain change at 480 eV loss. Two measurements, with different acquisition times, were used to generate this composite spectrum. (Bottom) EDX spectrum of the same sample in the same instrument (the Cu signal is due to the sample support grid).

with an EDX spectrum from the same sample. It can be noted that instead of the characteristic peaks of the EDX spectrum, steps or edges occur in the EELS spectrum. A complete description of EELS can be found in Egerton (1996).

8.4 Auger electron spectroscopy (AES)

AES can be used to identify the chemical composition and in some cases the chemical bonding near the surfaces of samples. The basic processes of Auger electron emission involve the production of an atomic inner shell vacancy by electron bombardment, and the subsequent decay of the atom from this excited state by the emission of an energetic electron, the Auger electron. As we explained in Chapter 2, this electron has a characteristic energy, which allows the identification of the emitting atom to be determined. AES has good spatial resolution, to approximately 20 nm, depending on the electron gun used, and can be used for compositional mapping. Typical sensitivity of Auger spectroscopy is of the order of 100 ppm, although it is not able to detect hydrogen and helium. Since it is a surface-specific technique, it is possible to perform depth profiling by using an ion beam to sputter material progressively from the surface of the sample, but this is destructive, of course. It requires an ultra-high vacuum system.

An important advantage in AES is the ability to determine chemical information using the shifts and shapes of the peaks of the Auger spectra. The ability to do depth-profiling makes Auger an important technique for thin film analysis, there being no real equivalent technique in EDX analysis, except cross-section analysis of thin films in the TEM.

Auger systems are available for SEM and TEM applications, but these systems lack the advantages of using an ultra-high vacuum system and combined ion beam sputtering systems. Auger analysis is particularly sensitive to low-Z elements, which have high Auger yields. Auger quantification relies on the use of standards in the same way as accurate quantitative EDX measurements.

Figure 8.4 shows a typical Auger spectrum.

8.5 X-ray photoelectron spectroscopy (XPS)

XPS, also known as ESCA, is another surface-sensitive technique which involves monochromic soft X-rays ejecting photoelectrons from the sample. The kinetic energy of the electrons identifies the elements present; small shifts in the energies provide additional chemical information. XPS can identify all elements except hydrogen and helium from depths from two monolayers to 25 monolayers (depending on the element).

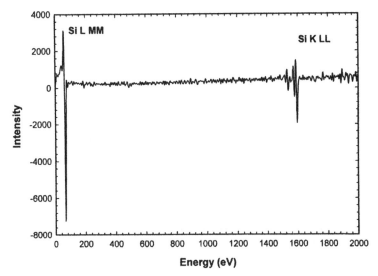

Figure 8.4. Typical Auger electron spectrum, obtained in a Physical Electronics 660 system, from a clean sample of pure Si (illustration courtesy of E. L. Shaw, MIT).

Subtle changes in the spectrum that occur as the sample is tilted can lead to information about the depth-distribution of the elements. Typically, XPS peak energies range between 500 and 1400 eV. XPS permits good quantification and good chemical state determination. Compared to EDX analysis its weaknesses are lack of spatial resolution (usually limited to about 70 μm) and moderate sensitivity at about 0.1 at%.

Figure 8.5 shows a typical XPS spectrum, compared to a TEM EDX analysis of the same material.

By far the major advantage of XPS is the ability to obtain chemical state information relatively easily. It is a surface technique that allows ready analysis of thin films and interfaces by depth-profiling, as in the Auger technique. Elemental concentrations can be determined with approximately the same accuracy as in EDX analysis.

8.6 X-ray fluorescence (XRF)

XRF uses an X-ray beam to excite characteristic secondary X-rays from the sample (the process was described in Chapters 2 and 3). The primary X-rays can be generated by a powerful X-ray tube or by a radioactive emitter. The detector can be a WDS or EDX system. The technique is non-destructive, quick and can be used quite effectively on bulk samples, which are not usually under vacuum. Typical applications include metals and archaeological samples, which require a non-destructive method of

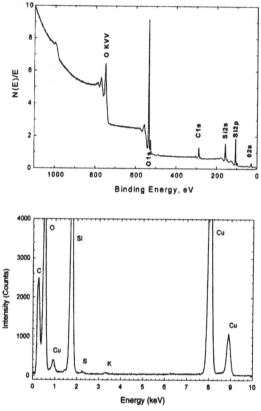

Figure 8.5. (Top) XPS spectrum from bulk sample of domestic gas burner soot. (Bottom) EDX spectrum of the same sample showing concentrations of Si and C (the Cu signal is due to the support grid) (D. C. Bell, L. C. Rainey, J. B. VanderSande, 1999).

analysis. Since the primary X-rays penetrate quite deeply into the sample, compared with electrons, another application is the measurements of moderately thin films and layer thicknesses.

A system including a radioactive primary excitation source and a portable EDX detector can be used to perform analysis of samples which cannot be taken into the laboratory – artwork often is analysed by this means, as curators are typically reluctant to allow pieces to be taken from museums. Another application would be extremely large samples, which are simply not portable.

XRF is well described in the literature, for example, see Jenkins (1974) and Bertin (1970). Analytical precision is usually listed as about 1%, with elemental detection limits of around 0.1%, depending on the surrounding matrix. Spatial resolution, on the other hand, is typically of the order of a millimetre, because of the difficulty of focusing the primary X-ray beam. These figures vary widely with the design of the system, though.

8.7 Atom probe

All the alternative analytical methods we have described so far have similarities to EDX analysis. There are many other, unrelated techniques, which we will not mention. One exception to this, though, is the atom probe.

In the atom probe, an extremely sharp point (or 'tip') made of the material under investigation is placed in a vacuum at high-voltage with respect to a detector. Because the sharp point concentrates the electric field due to the voltage, the field at the surface of the sample is extreme – of the order of several volts per nanometre. By careful adjustment, it is possible to arrange for the atoms of the tip to be 'dragged off' by the field (the process is called 'field evaporation'), and position-sensitive detectors measuring the time-of-flight of the atoms from the tip can determine their mass, and hence their identity, as well as where they were in the sample. Hence it can be accurately said that in the atom probe, the sample is taken apart, atom by atom, each one being individually identified. Surely this is the ultimate microanalytical technique!

There are, of course, limitations. Only samples that can be made into sharp tips can be examined. It can be very difficult to prepare samples so that the features of interest are in the observable volume, which is small because the tip radius increases as the material evaporates, until the field evaporation stops, or the voltage goes so high that an arc is generated, destroying the remaining sample. Even if a sharp point can be made, the electrostatic force on the tip can be so high that it yields and fails mechanically before field evaporation takes place.

However, in some applications, it is an invaluable tool, taking over at the limit of EDX analysis in the STEM to allow the investigation of samples in exquisite detail.

8.8 Overall strengths and weaknesses

EDX analysis is a highly effective technique for determining the elemental constituents of a sample, and can be used to derive chemical concentrations with reasonable accuracy, especially if there is a standard available. The ease of use, coupled with minimal operator training required, makes EDX an obvious choice for performing qualitative microanalysis; characteristic X-ray peaks are easily identified from available tables or software databases. The signal-to-noise in an EDX spectrum means that even without background subtraction realistic semi-quantitative information can often be derived from spectra.

EDX combined with an imaging system such as a TEM or SEM allows a spectrum to be obtained from a point in the image, which then relates chemical information to morphological details. The spatial resolution of EDX analysis is good, exceeded perhaps only by EELS and, of course, the atom probe, and X-ray mapping can form an image of elemental distributions in a sample. Samples for TEM investigation need to be thin but it is not necessary for them to be as thin as samples for EELS analysis, multiple scattering being less of an issue.

Once installed, the EDX system usually only requires re-calibration at infrequent intervals, unlike other microanalysis systems that require calibration before each sample analysis. Commercial EDX system vendors compete to provide easy-to-use software and systems that take on 'expert' ability, allowing the user to simply ask for particular information (the user should still understand the technique, since grave errors can be made by so-called 'expert' systems). EDX equipment is also typically relatively inexpensive compared to other analysis systems, and since it is only a small component of the budget required for a microscope system, is often easy to include in the complete purchase. Ease of use, low operator effort and the high accuracy of results makes EDX the technique of choice for a wide range of microanalysis problems.

Bibliography

It is not the purpose of this book to present an exhaustive bibliography. The sources listed here are of two types. The first five citations on the list include a few volumes that we recommend to our students as a way of expanding on the material we have presented in the present text. Of these, Goldstein *et al.* (1994) is almost the *de facto* standard reference of SEM imaging and microanalysis, while Joy *et al.* (1986) for a long time served the same function for the TEM microanalyst, although Williams and Carter (1996), presenting the material with less detail, but updated and in more readable form, also has much to recommend it. Heinrich *et al.* (1981) and Williams *et al.* (1995) are two compilations of conference papers, which, together, give a detailed account of the theory, operation and applications of the semiconductor X-ray detector. These volumes will lead the reader to other sources – at least as of their respective publication dates. For more recent developments, a good starting point would be papers presented in conferences, for example the annual proceedings of the Microscopy Society of America and the Microbeam Analysis Society (published together in recent years as part of *Microscopy and Microanalysis*, by Springer).

The remainder of the list includes the sources of specific details quoted in this book.

Goldstein, J.I., Newbury, D.E., Echlin, P., Joy, D.C., Romig, A.D., Lyman, C.E., Fiori, C. and Lifshin, E. (1994) *Scanning Electron Microscopy and X-ray Microanalysis*, 2nd Edn. Plenum Press, New York.

Joy, D.C., Romig, A.D. Jr and Goldstein, J.I. (1986) *Principles of Analytical Electron Microscopy*. Plenum Press, New York.

Heinrich, K.F.J., Newbury, D.E., Myklebust, R.L. and Fiori, C.E. (1981) *Energy Dispersive X-ray Spectrometry*, NBS Special Publication 604. US Department of Commerce, Washington, D.C.

Williams, D.B. and Carter, C.B. (1996) *Transmission Electron Microscopy: A Textbook for Materials Science*. Plenum Press, New York.

Williams, D.B., Goldstein, J.I. and Newbury, D.E. (Eds) (1995) *X-ray Spectrometry in Electron Beam Instruments*. Plenum Press, New York.

Bell, D.C., Rainey, L.C. and VanderSande J.B. (1999) Discrete single particle microanalysis of soots. *Air Pollution 99 Proceedings*, San Francisco, California.

Bertin, E.P. (1970) *Principles and Practice of X-Ray Spectroscopic Analysis*. Plenum Press, New York.

Brundle, C.R., Evans, C.A. and Wilson, S. (1992) *Encyclopedia of Materials Characterization*. Butterworth-Heinemann, Boston.

Carpenter, D.T., Watanabe, M., Barmak, K. and Williams, D.B. (1999) Low-magnification quantitative X-ray mapping of grain-boundary segregation in aluminum-4 wt% copper by analytical electron microscopy. *Microsc. Microanal.* **5:** 254.

Castaing, R. (1951) PhD thesis, University of Paris.

Chapman, J.N., Gray, C.C., Robertson, B.W. and Nicholson, W.A.P. (1983) X-ray production in thin films by electrons with energies between 40 and 100 keV. *X-Ray Spectrometry* **12:** 153, 163.

Chapman, J.N., Nicholson, W.A.P. and Crozier, P.A. (1984) Understanding thin film X-ray spectra. *J. Microsc.* **136:** 179.

Cliff, G. and Lorimer, G.W. (1975) The quantitative analysis of thin specimens. *J. Microsc.* **103:** 203.

Egerton, R.F. (1996) *Electron Energy-Loss Spectroscopy in the Electron Microscope*. Plenum Press, New York.

Fiori, C.E., Swyt, C.R. and Ellis, J.R. (1986) In: *Principles of Analytical Electron Microscopy*. (eds D.C. Joy, A.D. Jr Romig and J.I. Goldstein) Plenum Press, New York, p. 413.

Fiori, C.E., Swyt, C.R. and Myklebust, R.L. (1997) *Desk Top Spectrum Analyzer and X-Ray Data Base (DTSA)*. National Institute of Standards and Technology, Gaithersburg, Maryland.

Garratt-Reed, A.J. (1986) High resolution microanalysis of interfaces. *Mater. Res. Soc. Proc.* **62:** 115.

Hall, T.A. (1979) Biological X-ray microanalysis. *J. Microsc.* **117:** 145.

Heinrich, K.F.J. (1986) Mass absorption coefficients for electron probe microanalysis. *Proc. ICXOM XI*, London, Ontario, p. 67.

Jenkins, R. (1974) *An Introduction to X-ray Spectrometry*. Heydon, London.

Keyse, R.J., Garratt-Reed, A.J., Goodhew, P.J. and Lorimer, G.W. (1998) *Introduction to Scanning Transmission Electron Microscopy*. BIOS Scientific Publishers, Oxford.

Kramers, H.A. (1923) On the theory of X-ray absorption and of the continuous X-ray spectrum. *Phil. Mag.* **46:** 836.

Lechner, P., Eckbauer, S., Hartmann, R. *et al.* (1996) Silicon drift detectors for high resolution room temperature X-ray spectroscopy. *Nucl. Instr. Meth. A* **377:** 346.

Lowe, B.G. (1984) *Advances in Si(Li) Detector Technology – Series E Detectors*. Link Systems, High Wycombe.

Lund, M. (1995) In: *X-ray Spectrometry in Electron Beam Instruments* (eds D.B. Williams, J.I. Goldstein and D.E. Newbury). Plenum Press, New York, p. 21.

Marshall, D.J. and Hall, T.A. (1966) In: *X-ray Optics and Microanalysis* (eds R. Castaing, P. Deschamps and J. Philibert). Hermann, Paris, p. 374.

Moseley, H.G-J. (1913) The high frequency spectra of the elements, part 1. *Phil. Mag.* **26:** 1024.

Moseley, H.G-J. (1914) The high frequency spectra of the elements, part 2. *Phil. Mag.* **27:** 703.

Pint, B.A., Garratt-Reed, A.J. and Hobbs, L.W. (1998) Possible role of the oxygen potential gradient in enhancing diffusion of foreign ions on a-Al2O3 grain boundaries. *J. Am. Ceram. Soc.* **81:** 305.

Woldseth, R. (1973) *X-ray Energy Spectrometry.* Kevex Corp., Foster City, California.

Zaluzec, N.J. (1984) *A beginner's guide to x-ray analysis in the analytical electron microscope: Part 2 – Quantification using absorption and fluorescence corrections,* EMSA Bulletin 14(2):61.

Index

Printed in the United Kingdom
by Lightning Source UK Ltd.
102160UKS00002B/133-171

For Product Safety Concerns and Information please contact our EU
representative GPSR@taylorandfrancis.com Taylor & Francis Verlag GmbH,
Kaufingerstraße 24, 80331 München, Germany

Printed and bound by CPI Group (UK) Ltd, Croydon, CR0 4YY
01/05/2025
01858523-0001